T0358242

The Borderline Psychotic Child

The Borderline Psychotic Child reviews the history and evolution of the borderline diagnosis for children, in both the USA and the UK, bringing the reader up to date with current clinical opinion on the subject. Using a range of clinical case studies, the book attempts to harmonize US and UK views on borderline diagnosis in the light of new developments in theory at the Menninger Clinic, the Anna Freud Centre and the Tavistock Clinic.

Providing an introduction to the borderline concept, and a systematic overview of current theoretical thinking and clinical practices from leading practitioners in the field, *The Borderline Psychotic Child* will make informative reading for both professionals and students in the field of child analysis.

Trevor Lubbe trained as a child psychotherapist at the Tavistock Clinic, London, before returning to South Africa, where he now lives and works. He is founder editor of the journal *Psychoanalytic Psychotherapy in South Africa*.

The Borderline Psychotic Child

A selective integration

Edited by Trevor Lubbe

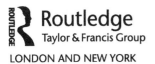

Routledge
Taylor & Francis Group

LONDON AND NEW YORK

First published 2000 by Routledge
2 Park Square, Milton Park, Abingdon, Oxon OX14 4RN
605 Third Avenue, New York, NY 10017

Routledge is an imprint of the Taylor & Francis Group, an informa business

Typeset in Times by Florence Production, Stoodleigh, Devon.

British Library Cataloguing in Publication Data
A catalogue record for this book is available from the British Library

Library of Congress Cataloguing in Publication Data
The borderline psychotic child : a selective integration / edited by Trevor Lubbe.
    p. cm.
  Includes bibliographical references and index.
  1. Borderline personality disorder in children.
    I. Lubbe, Trevor, 1952–

RJ506.B65 B68 2000
618.92′85852–dc21   99–048948

ISBN 13: 978-0-415-22219-8 (hbk)

DOI: 10.4324/9780203361153

Contents

PART II
Clinical challenges   107

Contributors

Anne Alvarez is a Principal Child Psychotherapist and co-convenor of the Autism Workshop at the Tavistock Clinic, London. She is a visiting professor in the Department of Child Neuropsychiatry at the University of Turin.

Robin Anderson is a Member of the Royal College of Psychiatrists and a child and adult psychoanalyst in part-time practice. He is chairman of the Adolescent Department at the Tavistock Clinic.

Efrain Bleiberg, MD, is President of the Menninger Clinic, Topeka, Kansas. He is a faculty member of the Karl Menninger School of Psychiatry and Mental Health Sciences where he teaches both child and adolescent psychiatric residents. He also serves as supervising and training analyst at the Topeka Institute for Psychoanalysis.

Peter Fonagy is Freud Memorial Professor of Psychoanalysis and Director of the Sub-department of Clinical Health Psychology at University College London. He is Director of Research at the Anna Freud Centre, London, and Director of the Child and Family Centre at the Menninger Foundation, Kansas. He is a clinical psychologist and a training and supervising analyst in the British Psycho-analytical Society. He is Vice-President of the International Psycho-analytical Association and is the current chair of its Standing Committee on Research.

Juliet Hopkins is a child psychotherapist on the staff of the Tavistock Clinic, London, who works within the independent tradition of British psychoanalysis. She is also an adult psychotherapist in private practice. She has particular interests in infant mental health, infant–parent psychotherapy and problems of parenting, and has published on these and related subjects.

Trevor Lubbe trained as a child psychotherapist at the Tavistock Clinic before returning to South Africa, where he now lives and works. He is a Member of the Association of Child Psychotherapists and a Member of the Cape Town Psychoanalytic Psychotherapy Study Group. He is Editor of the journal *Psychoanalytic Psychotherapy in South Africa*.

Lesley Pover is a child psychotherapist trained at the Tavistock Clinic, London. She is employed by the North East Essex Mental Health NHS Trust.

Beatrice Smith holds a degree in Art History and Mathematics as well as a Master's degree in Clinical Psychology from the Sorbonne, Paris. She was trained as a child psychotherapist at the Anna Freud Centre, where she currently works.

Mary Target is a senior lecturer in Psychology at University College London. She is a clinical psychologist and is currently training in adult psychoanalysis. She is Deputy Director of Research at the Anna Freud Centre.

Acknowledgements

I would like to thank Peter Fonagy for his encouragement when I first suggested to him the idea of this book. I am also grateful to him for his helpful suggestions and for allowing me such generous access to the libraries and computer facilities at University College London. To the authors I am grateful on three accounts – for their awkward questions about the topic, which helped me to clarify the aim and direction of this book, for the work they subsequently put into their chapters, and for the liberties they allowed me in editing their contributions. Margot Wadell read Chapter 1 and I would like to acknowledge her enthusiastic comments. Susan Budd was also very helpful in getting me to think about the overall shape and rationale of the book.

Further acknowledgements must be made to the following original sources from which material was reproduced or expanded for this book. Some of the material in Chapter 2 was first published by the author in the *Bulletin of the Menninger Clinic*, 58 (2), Spring 1994. A shortened version of Chapter 3 was presented by the authors as the 1997 Marianne Kris Memorial Lecture at the Annual Meeting of the Association for Child Psychoanalysis Inc., March 1997, Cancún, Mexico. Chapter 4 is an edited version of material which originally appeared in *Live Company* by Anne Alvarez, first published in Great Britain by Routledge in 1992. Copyright © 1992, 2000 Anne Alvarez. Reproduced by permission of the Author, c/o Rogers, Coleridge & White Ltd, 20 Powis Mews, London W11 1JN. Chapter 5, 'A case of foot and shoe fetishism in a 6-year-old girl' by Juliet Hopkins, was first published in *The International Review of Psychoanalysis* 11 (1984) and is reprinted by permission of the *International Journal of Psychoanalysis*. Chapter 6 contains 4 lines from 'Le Bateau Ivre' (p.65) in *Arthur Rimbaud: Collected Poems* translated by Oliver Bernard (Penguin Classics, 1962) copyright © Oliver Bernard, 1962. Reprinted by permission of Penguin Books Ltd. An earlier version of Chapter 9 appeared in *Psychoanalytic Psychotherapy in South Africa* 2 (1993).

Finally, I would like to take this opportunity of expressing my thanks to Ernst Freud who, all those years ago, introduced me to a totally new and fascinating type of observational method for studying infants at a time when the research tools I was using had taken me further and further away from the subject I was investigating – pre-term babies and their mothers. Due to this chance encounter I was drawn away from academic psychology towards a more psychodynamic model for understanding the psychopathology of everyday infancy. Then to Irma Brenman Pick I owe thanks for guiding me towards my training in child psychotherapy at the Tavistock Clinic and to Sydney Press for sponsoring my first four years there. To all my teachers and colleagues I owe a similar debt of gratitude, but to Sheila Miller in particular I am grateful for helping me through my training. In conclusion, I would like to express my deepest appreciation to Yolanda Glaser for always being in the background and for letting me discover how apparently disparate voices can be brought together in a harmonious way.

Foreword

Robin Anderson

This book is more original and pioneering than might first appear from its modest and descriptive title. As the title implies, Trevor Lubbe attempts, through his own contributions and his commissioning of chapters by other authors, to explore this difficult field of the borderline child. However, instead of ignoring versions that are too confusing or too different and settling for the definitions closest to his own preferred theoretical base, the editor has explored the wide field of different writers in North America and the United Kingdom, to extract the essence of their ideas. In order to pursue this approach, the editor has had to bear with the contradictions in the very different perspectives and viewpoints, a task which he says requires being able to tolerate feelings of being in a borderline state. However, this truly scholarly and sound exploration really does reap dividends because it has enabled him to do what so many workers in the field have failed to do, and that is to find what is valuable in the different approaches to psychoanalytic research and to look for common ground where the different findings can enhance each other rather than, as so often is the case, compete with each other for supremacy. In doing this, Lubbe in no way diminishes the genuine differences and sometimes fundamental disagreements which exist, but rather he makes clear that he is interested in what they can contribute to the central pool of knowledge.

Lubbe is particularly interested in bringing together the work of the many North American pioneers such as Mahler, Kernberg, Pine and Geleerd with the very clinically based work of the British object relations school, especially Klein and Winnicott. The recent work of Fonagy and Target, closely linked with the Anna Freud Centre in London, has been an important bridge between the work on the two sides of the Atlantic. Of particular interest is the way Lubbe has taken some of the very rich clinical contributions of the Kleinian school and drawn them into the debate, from which they have traditionally to some extent remained separated, probably both because of a deep and long-standing North American ambivalence to Kleinian ideas and because of a tendency among Kleinians to concentrate on developing their own ideas without entering into wider debates. It is interesting that Lubbe makes his attempt to draw them in at a time when there is a surge of interest in Kleinian ideas in the United States. Lubbe has shaped this book by surveying the wider field in considerable detail in the first chapter and then inviting theoretical contributions from four outstanding contributors to the field, setting out the views in North America and in the United Kingdom and then allowing the reader to reflect on these views in a series of clinical papers.

Finally, and not least important, Lubbe has made a contribution to the concept of childhood. The borderline child is not a step-child of the borderline adult. The findings that have led to this category are not extrapolations backwards from adulthood but a development which has come from psychoanalytic work with children.

Lubbe describes his book as a selective integration, but his selection is based on a deep consideration of what the different writers and schools have to say and taking the essence of each. In Bion's terms he has chosen the 'selected facts'. I think it is very interesting that this book is edited by a South African because its underlying philosophical approach is that if different groups can pool their contributions and contain their differences, the result is a richness that none of them can provide individually. This is an integrated book.

Preface

The appearance in 1983 of Kenneth Robson's edited collection entitled *The Borderline Child: Approaches to Etiology, Diagnosis and Treatment* was hailed at the time as a pioneering attempt to gather together the widely dispersed and disconnected data on this diagnosis for children. The contributors were mainly psychoanalytic practitioners seasoned in working with this client group, but by no means unaware of the classificatory dilemmas they present. Except for a few references by individual authors, no British or European contributions were included in the book. Strikingly, where such references were cited they were almost all theoretical, and this drew attention to the fact that psychoanalytical ideas developed in Britain had been highly influential in shaping the descriptive attempts by US clinicians to define borderline phenomena. Some notable examples were: Bowlby's attachment theories for Grinker *et al.* (1968); Fairbairn's 'split internalised bad object' and Winnicott's 'false self' for Rinsley (1980); Winnicott's 'mirroring' for Settlage (1977) and his 'transitional object' for Modell (1963); and Klein's 'ego splitting' and other primitive defence mechanisms for Masterson (1972) and Paulina Kernberg (1983a). These concepts proved felicitous to US clinicians and researchers in their deliberations about aetiology and diagnostic criteria – areas where British clinicians, ironically, would serve their own population of borderline youngsters less well, owing to a greater ambivalence within the child psychiatry community about the borderline concept and a less than enchanted attitude towards researching the subject.

In 1975 Gunderson and Singer referred to a growing 'provincialism' in the US literature owing to the sudden mushrooming of studies during the 1970s, which had caused a great scattering of the data. They specially chided authors whose inclination was to 'pay lip service to the previous literature [and to] proceed to describe borderline patients anew, without noting how their descriptions add to or simply repeat earlier contributions' (1975: 2). This, they claimed, had produced discrepancies and confusion in the literature, which they then set about surveying in order to identify those clinical features that were most commonly used in making this diagnosis. Eventually this practice itself, of surveying and trying to summarize the field as a whole, became a periodic feature of the literature – necessitated not so much by innovation as by the ever-expanding interest in this diagnosis which by the 1980s had reached its zenith. This included the child literature, too, and what Gunderson and Singer accomplished for the borderline adult in the 1970s other authors would do for the borderline child – Fred Pine in the 1970s, Vela, Gottlieb and Gottlieb in the 1980s, Petti and Vela, and Bleiberg in the 1990s. All were trying to co-ordinate and set this diagnosis within a new decade of research and clinical philosophy.

This brings the aim of the present book into focus. As we draw towards the end of the 1990s and approach a new century, there remains perhaps one outstanding synthesis that is yet to be reflected in the literature. This involves crossing the border between clinical psychoanalytic opinion in the USA and the UK with the intention of uncovering common ground and mutual influences. Moreover, an attempt to harmonize the views of different theoretical approaches within Britain itself is also lacking, especially in the light of refinements and advances in theory over the last decade. This is the aim of Chapter 1 of this book. The editor has keenly borne in mind the advice of Gunderson and Singer not to pass over too lightly the previous literature. Hence the approach of the first chapter will be to look in detail at how, historically, borderline children were first identified by child analysts in the USA and the UK. The purpose will be to show a convergence of clinical opinion which is the result of common beginnings and of facing common clinical uncertainties.

The remainder of Part I brings us into the present by showing developments in current theory at the Menninger Clinic, the Anna Freud Centre and the Tavistock Clinic and how these translate into practice. The concept of borderline disorders in children has always been controversial, and its emergence has been no less of a challenge to the coherence of theory, especially child theory.

How do we conceptualize a form of childhood disturbance that extends well beyond the infantile neuroses but which is not an unmistakable psychotic illness? In these chapters the reader will discover a shift in the theory of developmental pathology from the language of desire and conflict in object relations to a language of the mind – concepts concerning the growth of the mind, the pre-stages of such growth, the hidden potential for mental growth, as well as concepts describing forces that inhibit or impair mental stability and functioning. I believe this is where a great deal of convergence between different theoretical strands in psychoanalytic thinking can be found today, and Part II of the book illustrates these developments through several clinical case studies.

Part I

Crossing the borders

Current perspectives

Chapter 1

The borderline concept in childhood

Common origins and developments in clinical theory and practice in the USA and the UK

Trevor Lubbe

> It takes so little, so infinitely little, for a person to cross the border beyond which everything loses meaning: love, convictions, faith, history.
>
> Milan Kundera: *The Book of Laughter and Forgetting*
> (Penguin Books 1981)

Psychotic or psychotic-like features are found in a broad range of psychological disorders in childhood – in autism (and some of its subtypes), in childhood schizophrenia, in schizotypal disorder, and even some affective disorders. There are occasions too when a traumatic incident in childhood results in a transient reactive psychosis. When using the term 'psychotic', what psychoanalytic clinicians most frequently have in mind is a pattern of behaviour marked by a severe impairment to reality testing (A. Freud 1956; Rapoport and Ismond 1984). Children who exhibit such features appear to have made a qualified commitment to a reality independent of the self, but their integration with that reality remains incomplete.

When these features are observed in children who appear severely neurotic, the term 'borderline' or 'borderline psychotic' has been applied. The technical term 'borderline' was first used with children in the 1950s, roughly by analogy with features found in adults whose symptoms were seen as lying between the 'neurotic' and 'psychotic'. In children, the clinical picture was one in which symptoms clearly extended well beyond neurosis, yet they did not meet the criteria necessary for the diagnosis of childhood psychosis. Pre-eminent in this picture is the alternation between neurotic and psychotic functioning.

To date, many high-profile clinical studies and reviews have appeared in the child literature, mainly by psychoanalytic practitioners, outlining a distinctive pattern of symptoms associated with these 'in-between' disturbances, as Winnicott (1985) once described them. Vela *et al.* (1983), for example, identified a cluster of six main criteria – disturbed interpersonal relationships, disturbances in a sense of reality, excessive intense anxiety, impulsive behaviour, neurotic-like symptoms like rituals, obsessions and somatic concerns, and an early history of uneven or distorted development. However, because these symptoms do not constitute a clear-cut variant of the psychoneuroses, or the psychoses, there has been a great deal of disagreement and controversy about where precisely to place children who meet these criteria within a systematic diagnostic system.

According to Petti and Vela (1990), successive versions of the DSM have placed these children in two broad diagnostic spectra – the Schizotypal Personality Disorder/Autism/Schizophrenia spectrum and the Borderline Personality Disorder/Borderline spectrum. While such a variation in classificatory practice surely reflects how clinically confusing these children can be, it also clearly reflects a split among diagnosticians/researchers between those who favour placing them *inside* psychosis and those who view them as *outside* psychosis, but with so-called 'associated' or 'transitory' features. This has led to considerable diagnostic ambiguity, some authors emphasizing thought disturbances while others give more weight to object relations deficits; in fact, the above authors, while maintaining that their division is an arbitrary one and motivated principally by a desire to summarize the field as a whole, are nevertheless guilty of promoting this split by implying that psychotic features are found in the schizotypal spectrum only. This highlights another problem, namely, that many commentators today seem to address only the *manifest* behaviour of borderline children, and they shape their diagnostic thinking accordingly, without considering what lies underneath by way of mechanisms and structures.

It is certainly true that for the reviewer attempting to encompass the field as a whole, or for the researcher attempting a clinical communication or the replication of a study, the task is frequently bewildering – tantamount to comparing apples with pears or of having to face in several directions simultaneously – a somewhat 'borderline' experience in itself. Yet some of these problems of diagnostic ambiguity appear to stem directly from the uncritical use of psychiatric classification systems that draw sharp distinctions between psychotic and non-psychotic conditions, keeping them clearly delineated (Tarnopolsky *et al.* 1995). This practice reached its pinnacle in the ICD (International Classification of Diseases) 10 nomenclature, which contains no borderline diagnosis for children, and where evidence of atypical development is restricted to the diagnosis of a pervasive developmental disorder – without psychotic signs. Psychoanalytic practitioners would challenge this convention directly through their more elastic concepts of normality and psychopathology, which in some cases has led them to devise their own private definitions of what is 'psychotic' in order to represent the cognitive as well as object relations deficits in this group of children (Pine 1974; Kernberg 1975; Masterson and Rinsley 1975).

In this context it is worth mentioning Fred Pine's (1974; 1983) attempts to resolve some of the problems of diagnostic validity and specificity. Working within the classical nomenclature, he claimed to be satisfied that a 'borderline syndrome' could be identified in childhood with specific subtypes which have common aetiologies and common structures. He included children from both the psychotic border (schizoid personality) and the neurotic border (borderline) as subtypes – a broad and somewhat pragmatic view, but one that nevertheless tried to encompass the 'split' in diagnostic practice mentioned above which has generated so many inconclusive debates in the literature.

Pine (1983: 98) also mentions the importance of developmental factors in determining aetiology and in shaping therapy technique, and increasingly psychoanalytic clinicians are placing developmental factors at the heart of their deliberations. This is a significant point of departure, because it allows contemporary workers to base their arguments for diagnostic validity on data from developmental psychopathology research rather than on proving continuities with adult disorders, as in the past. The other advantage is that a developmental viewpoint provides a context in which both psychotic and non-psychotic symptoms can be accommodated diagnostically. Other attempts to find an accommodation have come from authors like Cohen *et al.* (1986) and Towbin *et al.* (1993) who have defined borderline disturbance as a 'multi-complex' developmental disorder. In this way they are able to include disturbances in thinking, as manifested in bizarre ideas, confusion of reality and fantasy, and delusions, etc., along with impairments in emotional regulation and social reciprocity, in their criteria for a 'borderline' diagnosis.

My aim in this chapter is to look back at the history of the borderline concept and to give an account of how this group of children were first identified by child psychoanalysts, and how their distinctive symptoms came to be classified within the different theoretical frameworks within our discipline, in both the USA and Britain. I believe it is worth examining this history in a little more detail than is nowadays customary. Contemporary writers, when referencing these early studies, tend to do so in a perfunctory way, as if they are of historical interest only. While history has certainly moved on – especially in recognizing the role of infant and child trauma and abuse in the aetiology of borderline pathology – it is striking how little that is new has been added to our understanding of these children from a descriptive or psychodynamic viewpoint. And yet equally striking has been the rather limited influence these remarkably fresh, pioneering studies have had upon current thinking and practice. In many ways the current profile of borderline youngsters, loaded down as it is with descriptions of conduct disturbance, attention deficit, impulsivity and emotional disregulation, is largely unrecognizable in the vivid but subtle descriptions of the early contributors, especially when detailing their primitive thought processes and difficulties in reality testing. It may well be timely, therefore, to remind ourselves of what was so compelling and unique about this group of children which had been uncovered for the first time within an analytic setting.

But my main purpose in looking at these early studies is to illustrate a common history, and to show how common clinical problems faced by child clinicians in the USA and the UK have led to a great deal of convergence around conceptual and technical issues. While it is obviously true that clinicians in North America and Britain, as well as those within Britain, differ sometimes reflexively in their allegiance to a particular theoretical framework within child psychoanalysis, it can nonetheless be shown from the clinical work with children of 'mixed psychopathology' that these differences are far outweighed by common understandings and common clinical stratagems, *especially when we take into account recent revisions in theory that have taken place within the mainstream child approaches in order to accommodate this group of children.*

Beginnings

The diagnosis and treatment of 'borderline' disorders in childhood by the psychoanalytic method has a long and acclaimed history which dates back to the early study and analytic treatment of psychotic children. Beginning in the 1930s in the UK, and 1940s in the USA, the 'case' for schizophrenia in childhood was strongly supported by many psychoanalytic clinicians, and the growing influence of their theories upon the general child psychiatry community became a striking feature in this area. The discovery of a new clinical syndrome – the 'deviational' or 'borderline' child – emerged largely as an offshoot of this research, and at the time this created a similar surge of scientific interest, as reflected in an ever-expanding literature, which according to some authors reached flood proportions in the 1980s. Psychoanalytic practitioners have continued to be active, not only in cataloguing and patrolling the borders of this specific disorder, but also in taking up the therapeutic challenges of working with this baffling and often acutely disturbed group of children.

One final comment on beginnings. In 1910, when Freud assessed the developmental history of the Wolfman, he puzzled over how, in his childhood, each libidinal stage was never properly succeeded by the one following it. Instead, each stage was left enigmatically side by side with all the others, and this allowed this boy to maintain an incessant vacillation, which in the end proved to be incompatible with the formation of a stable character. In 1974 Harold Blum claimed that the Wolfman's childhood was the first description of a borderline child in the psychiatric literature, and so it appears, yet again, that a small piece of metapsychology by Freud has successfully anticipated a whole quarry of psychoanalytic exploration.

USA

In the 1940s and 1950s several psychoanalytic studies were undertaken into the incidence of schizophrenia in small children and, while they did not start out as epidemiological studies, they were soon instrumental in establishing a nosological basis for differentiating a number of discrete conditions among psychotic children. In 1946 Elizabeth Geleerd was the first clinician to discern a subgroup of children who 'not always are considered psychotic' but who are in fact 'pre-psychotic', and who may go on to develop schizophrenia in adolescence. Her study drew upon the residents of Southward Residential School at the Menninger Clinic, and its findings were to set the frame for many generations of investigators both at this institution and at others throughout the USA. Geleerd drew attention to the incidence of grandiose fantasy and daydreaming in these children, to their lack of interest in their playmates, to their seclusiveness which became more entrenched with age. They gravitated, she noted, mainly towards adults, whose physical 'presence' and proximity helped to keep them alert and to some degree anchored to reality. At the time these observations were operationalized into a set of technical modifications for analytic work with the children: they had analytic sessions but it was believed that the transference effects of analysis could be maximized by assigning to each child a particular staff member, who would provide an actual relationship with the child by attuning himself or herself to the child's idiosyncrasies. Geleerd also highlighted the special quality of the anxiety in these children – 'free anxiety' she called it – which is not a signal of danger, as Freud had defined anxiety, but which marked out the helplessness of the ego in the face of id demands (1958: 294).

In a similar study at the James Putman Children's Center in 1949, Margaret Mahler and her colleagues also singled out a sample of children who fell at what they termed the 'benign' end of a continuum which led to more serious schizophrenic illnesses in childhood. These children employed primitive defences like fantasy formation, alteration between introjection and projection, and a type of 'mechanical' identification, but they also revealed sufficient ego organization to employ circumscribed neurotic-like defences, like rituals, obsessions and phobias, which operated in tandem with their scarred ego functioning. Their disturbance was viewed as an outcome of 'arrested development'.

Then in two pioneering papers Annemarie Weil (1953a; 1953b) identified a group of children whom she claimed 'hardly ever hit the middle line' (1953b: 523). By this she meant that they reacted always in extreme ways, and that their maturation on different levels had always been off-kilter. The clinical picture she compiled of them, particularly as they reached school age, was a remarkably vivid one and it became a classic in portraying the sorts of behavioural oddities characteristic of children at the so-called 'benign' end of the psychotic continuum. They played with words and neologisms, she said; they were 'restless', 'driven', and they 'wandered around' unproductively; they became 'overabsorbed' or 'compulsively centred on one object'; they were 'sensitive' but lacked interpersonal 'tact' and 'nuance'; they were either 'antagonistic' or showed a 'literalness in obeying authority'. She coined the term 'borderline' and described these children as a having a 'deviational *Anlage*' for the marked unevenness of their whole development which at all times had lacked integration.

By and large these early child studies in the USA had stressed a continuum of disturbance from candid psychosis to features close to, but not identical with, psychotic symptomology. Weil (1953a) and others predicted that their groups would eventually constitute a 'pool' from which acute forms of psychosis would later emerge. Dynamically, though, a different formulation was offered from that underlying adult psychosis. She claimed that the difficulties shown by these children were the result not of regression but of 'inadequate progression' (1953b: 528) and she viewed her work as supporting similar conclusions to those of Mahler. According to Mahler (1952), what distinguishes a malignant from a benign type of childhood psychosis is the stage of the ego's development where the psychotic break occurs. Weil (1970) developed her own concept of a 'basic core' – a fundamental layer which is established in the earliest weeks of life and with which the infant enters the symbiotic phase. A *damaged* 'core', she contended, is produced by disharmonies in the infant's constitutional makeup coupled with the mother's struggle with her attunements, which causes subsequent deviations in the child's maturational patterns, particularly in the child's capacity to form a balanced, harmonious relation to objects.

The application of the term 'borderline' or 'borderline psychotic' to children was not without its controversies, however, and some of these disputes remain active to this day – for example, the debate about whether borderline personality disorder exists in children under 12 (Kernberg and Shapiro 1990). In the early days many authors were unconvinced of the term's integrity and reliability as a discrete disease entity, and in view of its being at the 'border' of *existing* disease categories (i.e. neurosis and psychosis) they feared the term would simply become a fuzzy designation for miscellaneous forms of disturbance. Some argued that reliability could only be assumed if a continuity with adulthood versions of the disorder could be shown (Vela *et al.* 1983; Shapiro 1983).

In a series of papers Rudolf Ekstein and Judith Wallerstein (1954; 1956; 1957) cleverly reversed these arguments by claiming a diagnostic virtue for the fluctuating levels of ego functioning shown by these children. They argued that such was the fixed and predictable nature of these fluctuations that they justified the use of a distinct clinical category. For many clinicians this claim of a 'stable instability of ego functions' was to become an operational watchword for diagnosing these children, and hence for planning therapeutically for them. And it was but a short step on from this argument for other authors like Kernberg (1967; 1975) to claim that borderline symptomology reflects a level of ego deviance which is structural, and therefore sufficiently stable in its pathological effects to warrant the ascription of a personality disorder – a claim that was to have further significant implications for psychotherapy planning.

With the active clinician also very much in mind, Fred Pine's (1974; 1983) contributions have been important to present-day investigators. Struck by the ever-broadening domain to which the borderline diagnosis was being applied, he suggested that the way forward was to see the term not as a distilled category, but as a 'concept' which could be applied to general phenomena, in which there also existed variant forms – much like the 'concept' of the psychoneuroses. Pine saw the concept as applying to two broad areas of disturbance: to failures in crucial ego functions and to aberrations in object relations, with variations discernible in any one particular child. A 'working' nosology is how the author viewed the advantages of this approach, with gains accruing in clinical specificity.

Paulina Kernberg (1983a; 1983b) was another important contributor who has worked extensively with adolescents. She argued that the differences between the borderline child and adolescent flow from differences in developmental level only, and that the intrinsic psychopathology and the use of primitive defences was the same. Theoretically she also viewed the instability of the ego, or its weakness, in dynamic terms by linking them to excessive use of defensive manoeuvres. For example, like Otto Kernberg, she believed that, while projection typified the defensive repertoire of the neurotic patient, projective identification was the defence mechanism of choice for patients with borderline personality organization. She later compiled a very useful list of 31 defence mechanisms and divided them up according to their level of childhood psychopathology – normal, neurotic, borderline, psychotic (Kernberg 1994). On the whole, Kernberg has made her contributions with issues of treatment and technique in mind. While taking developmental considerations into account, her model is primarily a clinical one. For example, she has considered how ego defects and deficits in these children can be used actively for defensive purposes, for primary and secondary gains, to deal with frustration and anxiety (1983a: 115). She has also staunchly advocated the diagnosis of personality disorders in children under 12, including borderline personality disorder (Kernberg and Shapiro 1990), but contemporary clinical opinion in the USA remains divided on this question. The current situation is somewhat paradoxical: some authors contend that a developmental approach to child pathology naturally excludes considerations of personality (Shapiro 1990; Towbin *et al.* 1993) while others consider the concept of a personality disorder quite compatible with a developmental approach (Kernberg 1990; Bleiberg 1994).

Review of studies

Reviewing these early US contributions shows a clear development from the early studies of the 1940s and 1950s to the later ones of the 1960s and 1970s. Early authors were very much absorbed by the 'strangeness' of these borderline children, with their 'skinlessness'. As original writers, their interest was drawn towards their psychotic-like features and the lamentable restrictions which these features placed upon their lives. Their way of understanding the children's difficulties was in terms of deficit, limitation, developmental arrest. They were content, too, to use impressionistic language – words like 'baffling', 'peculiar', 'strange', 'odd' and 'bizarre' commonly appeared in their descriptions.

In the 1960s and 1970s the tone of the literature changed dramatically, when the focus shifted to the question of classification and related secular themes: criticisms of the breadth of childhood problems being labelled borderline; the question of continuities with the adult version of the disorder; questions of co-morbidity with other disorders; and other controversial issues such as whether or not the developmental and clinical features found in this group could be theorized as reflecting a personality disorder. Another important aspect of classification took place within psychoanalytic theory itself. This involved attempts to integrate these new discoveries, reflective of the widening scope of indications for child analysis, within existing theoretical systems, notably the theories of Anna Freud and developmental ego psychology theory. Margaret Mahler's pioneering work with psychotic children would provide the balance between the traditionalist impulse to modify or adapt existing theory and the need for fresh concepts.

The Kernberg school, the main proponent of the personality disorder position within adult psychopathology, would contribute in no small measure to advances in clinical child theory, and so set the stage for psychotherapy approaches aimed at specific ego-related pathology. But opponents have called into question whether the forging of a diagnostic category for children by analogy to an adult disorder has been an unqualified success (Shapiro 1983; Lofgren *et al.* 1991). These authors have been sceptical about whether diagnostic criteria for a personality disorder can ever be based on precise ego pathology without being blatantly theory-specific, in which case a focused therapeutic technique designed to undo this pathology, however successful, merely confirms a theory, not a diagnosis (Shapiro 1983). In today's world of competing concepts of psychopathology it remains doubtful whether *any* diagnostic system can be entirely theory-free, but what is striking about these criticisms is the way they echo the kind of objections made about Melanie Klein's clinical theories in the USA, namely, that they blurred the boundaries between metapsychological and clinical concepts so that they could never be proved or disproved. That the Kernberg school should be taken to task on similar grounds is ironic, given the extent to which Otto Kernberg fought shy of incorporating, without expurgation, the full logic of Melanie Klein's clinical theories.

United Kingdom

Work with children showing clinical signs of psychosis began in 1929 with Melanie Klein. By introducing acutely neurotic children to an analytic setting, she found that severe mental defects, hitherto hidden from adult attention, were uncovered, and that these defects were particularly in the areas of the children's capacity to play and in their relation to reality. Her conclusion was that schizophrenia in childhood was a more common illness than had previously been understood. In addition, the notion of *infantile psychosis* was developed to account for the paranoid substratum underlying what appeared in many children as gravely neurotic symptom formations. This concept of infantile psychosis was to occupy a central place in Kleinian formulations on psychopathology in general, and would provide the theoretical framework for a 'serial' concept of mental illness whereby a neurotic disorder, for example, could be seen as serving as an alibi for an underlying psychotic disturbance.

Initially Klein followed the grain of Karl Abraham's (1924) nosological method of ascribing specific fixation points: schizophrenia in childhood, she contended, was based on a regression to an oral-cannibalistic fixation. This was a clinical finding which in fact differed from Abraham's own verdict, which linked schizophrenia in adulthood to an oral sucking fixation, but Klein claimed she had based her conclusions on actual child data.

Turning to her earlier findings, with children showing a correlation between anxiety and learning inhibitions (Klein 1923), she now began to describe the clinical picture of the psychotic child's disturbance less in terms of a regression of the ego to its narcissistic origins, and more along the lines of a blocking of development owing to the ego's over-hasty and ineffective defences against sadism. In superabundance, she argued, these defences check the establishment of a relation to reality and to the development of fantasy life (1930a). This was an original theory, and in it we can see that her thinking followed the direction of a developmental arrest model rather than a regression model. The result was that the need for a nosological method quickly gave way to an emphasis on the specific character of the ego's defensive manoeuvres. Fixation, as a concept, was applied microanalytically to drive/ego configurations themselves and not to circumscribed developmental phases, and the precariousness of the ego, which is so characteristic of the infantile psychoses, was viewed not as a cause but as a consequence of the excessive use of defensive activities themselves. It was principally on this basis, i.e. on the basis of the economics of ego defences, that Klein eventually drew distinctions between infantile neurotic and psychotic symptomology, as well as a distinction between the childhood paranoiac and schizophrenic psychoses – in the paranoiac psychoses, she claimed, a projective relationship with reality dominates while in the schizophrenic psychosis there is a pathological denial of reality and a withdrawal into the world of fantasy (Petot 1990: 218).

Now these formulations greatly influenced the general approach to child analytic work within the Kleinian model. As I have indicated, the focus on the quality of anxiety and the economics of primitive defensive manoeuvres made it less compelling for clinicians to classify childhood disturbance along the lines of distinctive clinical traits or maladaptive behaviour, as exemplified in a psychiatric diagnostic system. The concept of 'states' was preferred to the concept of 'traits', and theoretically this meant that issues of psychic processes and mechanisms were kept quite separate from categories of disorder. Similarly, the notion of axes (vertical or horizontal) was applied exclusively to the structuralization of the child's defences, while methods of categorization were largely descriptive and dynamic, and pursued by differential diagnosis (Meltzer 1967). Then there was the concept of *infantile psychosis* which, as I have indicated, postulated the continuity of psychotic and non-psychotic states in every person. This concept was to find its most natural clinical expression in Bion's (1957) distinction between the psychotic and non-psychotic portions of every personality.

Clinically speaking, there were both gains and losses in this approach. One well-known spin-off was a less pejorative attitude towards disturbed behaviour in children, with the result that many children entered analysis who would otherwise have been considered inappropriate or even inaccessible to analytic work. As has been well documented, this led to refinements in child technique and at the same time stimulated new understanding around the origins of severe adult psychopathology (Segal 1979). What was overlooked, however, was a more varied and systematic evaluation of the non-psychotic spectrum, of the differences between normal, neurotic and psychotic, and of the developmental role of assets and deficits in all three areas.

Another obvious drawback was that this approach largely exempted Kleinians from the burgeoning debate in the child literature about the validity of diagnostic categories and the importance of a reliable nomenclature for children – nowadays a more pressing requirement in a world of diagnostic-based child psychotherapy supported by clinical outcome research. In fact, until the 1980s the term 'borderline' rarely appeared in scientific papers by Kleinian child therapists, even though the clinical descriptions of the children treated would clearly warrant such a diagnosis (Lush 1968; Tustin 1978; Trowell 1981; Hughes 1988). Where the term was applied to children, it was largely used as a spatial metaphor to indicate a distinct level of psychic functioning. As a result some important early contributions by Kleinians to this field have not penetrated mainstream psychoanalytic thinking.

Meltzer (1986), for example, delineated three non-autistic types of infantile psychosis based on separate developmental histories: failures of post-natal adjustment, primary failure of mental development, geographical confusional psychosis. He placed borderline disorders in the latter category, for which he defined a distinct genetic-dynamic pathway: a non-traumatic caesura followed by a passionate invitation from the mother for emotional contact. This invitation, however, is later withdrawn, leaving the infant with no means of comprehending this situation other than through premature phantasies of intrusion, culminating in a number of claustrophobic and agoraphobic reactions which are highlighted when the child enters pre-school or school. As a genetic-dynamic proposition this bears a close resemblance to some aspects of Mahler's (1971; Mahler *et al.* 1975) aetiologic formulations, which have been so influential for American writers on borderline pathology like Masterson and Rinsley (1975) and Kernberg (1967).

In the 1980s and 1990s the situation corrected itself, with the term 'borderline' appearing with greater frequency in publications by Kleinian child therapists, and this was mainly due to the writings of Alvarez (1985; 1989; 1992). The term, however, remains little used diagnostically because the emphasis by Kleinian therapists is still primarily a clinical one, that is, one that spotlights mental operations and mechanisms which in the child have become clustered into a defensive organization which acts as a safeguard against specific anxiety-generated conflicts (Steiner 1979; Jackson 1985). Steiner has theorized (from adult work) that these defensive organizations act as a substitute for a person's faltering attempts to negotiate anxieties associated with a depressive position, which leaves the individual functioning on the 'border' between the paranoid and schizoid positions. However, Alvarez (1985; 1992) examined the role of these defensive organizations in children more closely, and found that where the child suffers from severe psychic impoverishment the use of primitive defences may be less for the purposes of fortification and more as a 'proving ground' – which indicates an awakening or a discovery and not a retreat from reality. A careful evaluation of the ego, she contended, especially concerning its balances and imbalances, assists the clinician in deciding whether defensive or developmental considerations are paramount. These formulations, reflecting mainly technical concerns, went some way towards retrieving the *developmental* dimension to the Kleinian theory of the paranoid-schizoid position, and also had the benefit of reclaiming portions of child theory from those writers who have based their theoretical contributions principally on work with adults.

Winnicott

Winnicott similarly viewed the clinical picture of borderline disturbance in children in terms of a sophisticated defensive organization which he claimed was always an 'organisation towards invulnerability', that is, towards creating a suffering-free zone that insures against traumatic anxieties relating to experiences of early environmental failure (1967a). These organizations, he said, find their apotheosis in the autistic child, who achieves total invulnerability from suffering. The autistic child, he wrote, while not free of pain, is certainly free of suffering – because it is the parents who suffer.

It is important to stress that for Winnicott these failures were not failures in maternal provision alone, but they include as aetiological factors the actions of parents whose love and caring for their child were all reaction formations. That is, he took into account the parents' repressed hatred of the child – what lies behind the parents' eyes – in his assessment of the type of environmental failure that contributes to borderline states (Winnicott 1969). Along with actualized hatred, this factor now occupies a central place in contemporary thinking about borderline pathology, and in America it has been given a sophisticated clinical paradigm by Rinsley (1980) in his work with borderline adolescents.

Winnicott used the term 'borderline' at several points in his writings, referring to both child and adult cases. He worked with some cases in long-term psychotherapy and with other cases in management (Winnicott 1985), and though he never devoted a complete paper to the subject he did offer a definition:

> By the term 'borderline' I mean the kind of case in which the core of the patient's disturbance is psychotic, but the patient has enough psycho-neurotic organisation always to be able to present psycho-neurotic or psycho-somatic disorder when the central psychotic anxiety threatens to break through in crude form.
>
> (1968: 219–20)

According to Winnicott, the type of anxiety referred to here, though acute, implies some degree of integration and takes the form of 'falling forever', 'going off in all directions', 'loss of directed relating to objects', 'somatic split: head and body'. In borderline children – the 'in-betweens', as he depicted them – Winnicott looked to developmental factors to explain aetiology: the child has made a reasonable start in life but the experience of early environmental trauma, as distinct from deprivation, has caused prominent distortions in the maturational process (1967a; 1985). Where defensive organizations are in evidence, he stated, this usually implies that some secondary gains have established themselves within the personality which serve as a hedge against frank psychosis. Yet these secondary gains can, and must, be distinguished from those reflected in the hardened 'attitude' of antisocial types, which usually crystallize into delinquency – an important difference that has implications for therapy.

Several authors working with children have found Winnicott's ideas useful technically, particularly on the 'management' of borderline cases. Arnold Modell (1963) defined borderline pathology as a developmental disorder which has its origins in an arrest at the stage of the transitional object. Similarly, Finzy (1971) described a child whose prolonged relationship with a transitional object in early childhood became generalized to a transitional style of relating to all subsequent objects, which enabled him to appear normal outside therapy while in the sessions there was clear evidence of borderline psychotic features. Kernberg (1983a) also drew attention to the deviational history of transitional objects in borderline youngsters. Woods (1982) utilized a pre-interpretative 'holding' phase in therapy where the child's omnipotent denial of separateness from the therapist was not challenged until this could be tolerated. Finally, on a theoretical level Winnicott's ideas have been widely used by many authors contributing to the general field of borderline pathology, particularly in the USA – 'mirroring' by Settlage (1977), 'false self' by Rinsley (1980), 'transitional object' by Modell (1963) and Paulina Kernberg (1983a).

Anna Freud

From her earliest writings Anna Freud (1945) had always reserved a special constellation for thinking about those children whose problems were not reflected within the framework of an infantile neurosis but were recognizable by certain extreme distortions, impairments or disharmonies in their development. Her appreciation of what she termed 'developmental disturbance' grew over the years and with it her recognition of the technical adjustments required in the treatment of these children – though her acceptance of 'non-analytical' methods was always tempered by due considerations for true analytic goals and efficacy (Edgecombe 1995).

In her 1956 paper on the assessment of borderline children she characterized evidence of atypical development in terms of an excessive lag between drive, ego and superego development – a picture of disproportionality that she claimed typified the borderline child. In this paper she emphasized the diagnostic benefit of qualitative as well as quantitative factors in the appraisal of anxiety, object cathexis, ego boundaries and thought processes. The borders between 'neurotic' and 'borderline' were drawn quite sharply, but the 'mixed' nature of borderline pathology was confirmed through the deployment of both developmental and conflict considerations – the child's developmental impairments were seen as reflecting a deficit that was due to arrest, while the neurotic part of the personality could be subject to regressions, some of a possibly permanent nature. In terms of object relating, the child was seen as constantly on the border between object cathexis and primary identification, shuttling back and forth between an object-related stance and a merger with the object. Technically, however, sharp distinctions were upheld on what could be therapeutically optimal in working with this group of children – Anna Freud found the idea of interpreting conflict and defence deeply counterintuitive, and she consistently favoured what became known as the developmental 'by-products' of analysis as the technique of choice. These by-products included intimacy with the therapist as a new object, recognizing developmental anomalies and imbalances through verbalization, the use of reassurance, and correctional emotional experience for the purposes of spurring on confinements in development (Edgecombe 1995). Over time the validity of these 'by-products' would be tested, expanded and refined.

To define with greater precision the meaning of the borderline concept and to consider, from direct clinical evidence, the implications for child technique, a treatment study of 10 children of different ages was undertaken by Rosenfeld and Sprince and colleagues at the then Hampstead Clinic (1963; 1965). Through their Study Group they pooled their findings, adding some fresh outlines to the clinical picture current at that time: the role of primary identification in weakening object relations, the lack of Oedipal development across all ages with a clear fixation at the oral level, and the spontaneous outflow of fantasy material due to defects in repression. Primary identification refers to a merger of parts of the self with characteristics of the object – a primitive defence that utilizes an interpersonal context but nevertheless affects the intactness of the ego. At the time, however, it was to be the observed defects in repression, and not early defences of an interpersonal nature, that was to influence their principal recommendation on technique: interpretation of content, while perhaps relatively effortless for the therapist, should be avoided in the early phases of treatment until certain defences are better organized in the child. Anna Freud (1965) echoed these concerns by stating that the borderline child often 'misuses' interpretations by weaving them into the flow of anxiety-arousing fantasies – he 'uses the opportunity to turn the relationship with the analyst into a kind of *folie à deux*' (1965: 231). That this type of 'misuse' of the object might itself be the product of a set of dysfunctional self- and object-representations, expressed interpersonally, was only later to be linked to borderline disturbance (Rosenfeld 1972).

At present, 'developmental psychotherapy' is how contemporary workers at the Anna Freud Centre describe their approach to children with 'mixed psychopathology' (Fonagy and Target 1996a; Hurry 1998). To accomodate these children within a general theory of psychopathology Anna Freud's concept of a twin-track aetiological pathway (conflict and developmental) for childhood disturbance has been given a more explicit theoretical framework. Two models are proposed. First, there is a mental *representational* model where disturbance is reflected in compromise formations because of the exclusion of representations from consciousness – the 'classical' psychoanalytic view of psychopathology. In this model psychic change is effected via insight-orientated techniques (interpretation of conflict and defence) which achieve a better integration of conscious and unconscious representations. Then there is a mental *process* model which depicts disturbance as an *inhibition* or *disavowal* of mental processes resulting in a variety of developmental deficits. Therapeutic change comes about through 'developmental psychotherapy' – a flexible method which employs a range of techniques to remove inhibitions and to restore to children their mental capacities, optimally their capacity for self- and object-representations (Fonagy *et al.* 1993). Problems besetting borderline children and their treatment are dealt with within the terms of this model.

These developments place a clear focus on the mental functioning of the borderline child as it impacts on *interpersonal* reality (Fonagy 1991; 1995; Target and Fonagy 1994b). Citing evidence from cognitive psychology and social cognition studies, these authors highlight specific relational problems that stem from defects in the child's capacity to uphold or sustain a mental model of self-and-other relationships. Such a model allows the child to denote feelings, beliefs, desires to others and to him or herself; this capacity to 'mentalize' is a developmental acquisition which is based on the child's experience of having his or her own mental states reflected by the parents. In not being able to label their own mental states, or to attribute states of mind to others, these children demonstrate a flawed 'theory of mind', the evidence for which is to be found in repetitive interpersonal enactments that supplant emotional experiences that cannot, or cannot yet, be represented psychologically. Essentially this is a mental model approach to borderline disturbance with a social-learning theory underlay. Therapeutically, the goal is to recover underutilized mental functions; the emphasis is placed on mental processes and states, and on small changes in these states, which are pointed out to the child as they manifest themselves with the therapist and in references by the child to outside relationships.

Convergent themes

This survey of developments in the USA and the UK, and developments within the UK itself, makes it possible to discern several areas of diversity in discovery and conceptualization, but also allows a great deal of mutual understanding, which is surely the result of clinicians facing similar technical problems. My interest is in achieving a 'selective integration' (Mitchell 1988), and to this end I will be drawing out some unifying themes that have surfaced during the course of this survey.

History

It has been commonly asserted that the borderline concept in childhood appeared as an outgrowth of diagnostic considerations concerning the borderline adult – that it was the 'step-child' of investigations into the adult version of the disorder (Kestenbaum 1983; Massie and Rosenthal 1984). This is not true. In both the USA and the UK the growth point historically for a category of children with symptoms characterized as 'borderline' was psychoanalytic work undertaken with psychotic children. This is not to belittle the contribution of adult concepts and research to child versions of the disorder, but it is far from certain whether these influences have been felicitous, especially when we take into account the cost to diagnostic accuracy for children when stark developmental disparities with grown-ups are discounted (Shapiro 1983; 1990). *Per contra*, the theoretical and technical yield from this early analytic work with psychotic children was eagerly absorbed by clinicians working in the area of severe adult pathology.

The 1940s and 1950s were ebullient and progressive times for child analysis, and this can be keenly sensed in the formative papers of the day. The clinical work initially took centre-stage, and the theory was to follow, with new concepts coming into being to accommodate the discoveries made within the widening scope of indications for child work. Taking a global view, the influence of Anna Freud's contributions to our understanding of atypical development, together with the pioneering work with psychotic children by Melanie Klein and Margaret Mahler, supplemented by important concepts provided by Winnicott, were to set the framework internationally for defining borderline pathology throughout the psychoanalytic community and beyond.

Anxiety

There is a remarkable degree of convergence among all the major contributors about the role of anxiety, and its 'specialness', as a central symptomological feature of the borderline child (Klein 1930b; Geleerd 1946; 1958; Mahler *et al.* 1949; Weil 1953a; 1953b; Anna Freud 1956; Rosenfeld and Sprince 1963; Kernberg 1983a; Masterson 1972; Pine 1974; 1983; Steiner 1979; Alvarez 1985; 1992). While those authors influenced by Kleinian thinking frequently make reference to the theoretical role of anxiety in the child's personality, they nevertheless view anxiety as a prominent affect in this group of children – in both latent and manifest forms.

Geleerd (1958) claimed that this unique form of anxiety was in itself diagnostic, as it *differentiated* the psychotic from the borderline child. 'Free anxiety' she called it, and she contended that this was not a signal to a danger type of anxiety but was 'in the nature of a traumatic anxiety in the face of relatively mild frustrations' (1958: 294). Weil (1953b) too referred to the prominence of 'primitive anxiety' in her group of children. In their sample Rosenfeld and Sprince (1963) also found evidence of a failure to experience anxiety as a danger signal, which left the child vulnerable to panic states associated with intense feelings of disintegration and annihilation. They coined the term 'borderline anxiety' or 'world-catastrophe anxiety' to indicate its psychotic-like quality. Pine (1974) suggested that when the child is overwhelmed by this type of frantic anxiety a series of secondary defences are set in train which are highly successful in moderating anxiety – though they correspondingly undermine certain ego functions.

What is being identified here is the pivotal role that intense anxiety plays in the child's attempts to conduct normal object relations. A preponderance of anxiety drives the child towards the object and simultaneously away from it. Anna Freud (1956) suggested that such children are constantly on the border between object cathexis and identification. They may approach the object via primary identification but soon fear becoming engulfed, while the partial object cathexis that is the result inevitably leads to an abiding dread of being dropped at any moment. Other authors, like Masterson (1972), have described this type of anxiety-based shuttling in children's object relations in terms of Mahler's theory of separation–individuation.

Kleinian authors, backed up by their tradition of giving anxiety a central role in the formation of early defences (Klein 1935), use the term 'psychotic anxiety' to describe this situation. In truly psychotic children, of course, anxiety is conspicuous by its absence, which usually directs the clinician towards their defensive set-up, where the evidence for psychotic functioning is to be found. In borderline children where there is some ego development, a combustible cycle of concerns is observed about the safety of the self (persecutory anxiety) and the safety of the object (depressive anxiety). In addition, moving from depressive to persecutory anxiety and back again can become established as a fixed structure that can assume the significance of a defensive organization (Steiner 1979). This description resembles the metaphor used by Ekstein and

Wallerstein (1954) of an 'unreliable thermostat' to convey a sense of the child's vulnerability to ego-state fluctuations. 'We have suggested that patients in the borderline group seem to face absolute dilemmas which admit of no solution' (1954: 551).

Fantasy

Since Geleerd (1946) first described the profusion of 'omnipotent fantasies' in her group of children, this has been a feature stressed by all the major contributors. Mahler *et al.* (1949) placed fantasy formation alongside histrionics as examples of tertiary defences which replace the delusions of the more candidly psychotic child. Highlighted by both Weil (1953a) and Rosenfeld and Sprince (1963) was a marked defect in repression in these children, which they noted led to fantasy material being presented in an unguarded way – a frequently disquieting experience for the therapist. For Ekstein and Wallerstein (1954) the shift between contact with the therapist and retreat to idiosyncratic fantasy was a hallmark of the fluctuating ego states so much in evidence in their study. In the main, the concept of fantasy being referred to in these studies is not its usual sense, that is, of 'make-believe' or as a defensive denial of reality. Fantasy here refers to a defect in the ego which allows undistorted id-derivatives to intrude in such a way as to leave the child with a precarious grip on reality. Geleerd (1949) suggested that when the child gets caught up in fantasy the therapist should adopt a friendly, 'soothing' approach which strengthens his or her hold on reality. The therapist might also enter into the production of the child's fantasies as a means of modifying their content – a somewhat radical idea at the time but one that anticipates what clinicians would later recognize as the interpersonal dimension to the borderline child's defensive system.

Where fantasy does serve as a denial of reality or as unconscious wish-fulfilment is when it becomes woven into an enactment. Chethik and Fast (1970) described how the enactment of fantasy recruits another person into a particular role, which is designed to reinforce a distortion in reality the child is seeking to retain. While this type of enactment is described in terms of a narcissistic manoeuvre, the authors emphasize its developmental potential – an external object is, in fact, needed in order to actualize the fantasy. By a different route Kleinian therapists have reported that such enactments are brought about through the *phantasy* of projective identification, also a narcissistic manoeuvre involving omnipotent motives, particularly when it operates as an interpersonal defence against separateness (Rosenfeld 1964). When motivated by desperation and not purely by omnipotence, projective identification can also express a developmental need (Bion 1959).

Obsessional mechanisms

Another striking consensus exists around the prevalence of ritualistic and obsessional traits in borderline children. Unlike their role in neurotic children, as a defence against unthinkable thoughts or impulses, in borderline children obsessional mechanisms act as a hedge against unthinkable anxieties about disintegration and collapse. Weil (1953a; 1953b) frequently observed how children in her study became compulsively centred on one activity or one person. Frank psychosis is avoided, she noted, if the child channels his or her hostility into obsessional and ritualistic traits by which, too, a superficial socialization can be achieved. Geleerd also referred to the drive fusion aspect of obsessional symptoms, and obsessional defences were observed by Rosenfeld and Sprince (1963) in their study – who, like Weil, felt they were useful to the child. Masterson (1972) also identified obsessive-compulsive traits as a prominent feature of the clinical picture here.

Kleinian authors too have identified a similar role for obsessional mechanisms in even more profoundly psychotic children. In Meltzer *et al.*'s (1975) study on infantile autism, for example, certain defence mechanisms in autistic children were found to have features and aims in common with general obsessional mechanisms, principally the aim of 'simplifying' any emotional experience that would otherwise overwhelm the child. In autism these mechanisms render such emotional experiences meaningless by dispersing them into the perceptual conscious system of the body, the skin or the sense organs, with one dramatic result that the difference between animate and inanimate is eliminated. In borderline children, where the distinction between animate and inanimate endures and where an object cathexis exists due to some ego development, these obsessional mechanisms are most active when separation anxieties threaten integration. Bodily expressions of emotion, mechanical actions, ritualistic thinking are the means of 'simplification' in this diagnostic group (see Chapter 8).

Splitting

Prominent among the libidinal anomalies observed by Rosenfeld and Sprince (1963) in their sample of children was a faulty relationship between the drives and ego – they develop independently, they stated, 'as if they belonged to two different people' (1963: 615). Ekstein and Wallerstein (1954) noted further that rapid alterations in ego states were caused 'autistically', that is, by factors entirely endogenous to the child. With these findings in mind, it should not be surprising that the presence of primitive defence mechanisms has been emphasized by many authors in discussing borderline disturbances – omnipotence, idealization, denial, undoing, alteration of projection and introjection, primary identification, withdrawal into fantasy – and particularly splitting.

Masterson (1972) identified splitting as a key psychodynamic factor in borderline states and he also singled out excessive 'object splitting' as contributing expressly to the partial integration of the ego. Similarly, Pine (1983) refers to 'splitting of good and bad images of self and other' that results in dissociated mental states which tend to become activated in a split transference. What these authors are describing is how splitting safeguards the ego by keeping apart contradictory self- and object-representations, but they are also underscoring the damaging repercussions upon ego states and ego integration. Kernberg (1983a) notes that splitting takes over when repression is faulty in order to deal with the profusion of fantasy material as described by Weil (1953a) and Rosenfeld and Sprince (1963). But such failures, she argues, which imply a lack of early differentiation and structure, do not rule out a structured use of primitive defences, including splitting, idealization and devaluation.

While Kleinian therapists have emphasized splitting as a normal response of the immature ego facing early anxiety constellations, they distinguish this from the type of splitting that accompanies pathological projective identification, which is disintegrative by virtue of fusing parts of the ego with the object (Klein 1946). A breakdown in normal splitting is the result, which is substituted by a new defensive manoeuvre that involves the employment of an external object as a representative of the self for the performance of ego functions.

Winnicott (1952) had his own unique way of describing the results of splitting upon the borderline psychotic self. He claimed it was environmental failure that starts the individual off with a paranoid potential because it produces a basic split between the child and the environment. When the relation to the object is excessively depersonifying, then a cathexis to the self is conducted surreptitiously for the purposes of self-cohesion. In borderline cases, he stated, the split is enhanced through more and more defensive manoeuvres aimed at neutralizing environmental impingements – the result being an example of 'organized introversion'.

Defensive organizations

Placed as they are in a border region between neurosis and psychosis, this group of children presents us with striking examples of a plurality of defences, reflecting fluctuations between primitive, less primitive and precocious mental modes. These defences may become organized into defensive amalgams – the product of these fluctuations. If ever it was true that the choice of psychological illness is really a question of defensive preference, then borderline psychotic children, with their unique combination of defences, would exemplify this statement. What also needs to be borne in mind, however, is the cost to the children of the upkeep of these defensive systems.

There is unanimity among clinicians from different theoretical orientations about the instability of defences, the failure of defences and their replacement by organized systems of defence. Of course, by their nature defences, particularly primitive ones, do not operate in isolation and they enjoy a degree of improvisation and collaboration, but by 'defensive organizations' is meant a cluster of defences acting in concert in a dedicated way. Such organizations tend to establish themselves as alternative structures in the personality and in this way ego growth is compromised and development narrowed or brought to a standstill. Citing the case of mutism, for example, Pine (1974) claimed that the ego limitation seen in borderline children is directly linked to their 'heavily relied-upon defence organisations' that have evolved adaptively. In addition he describes the shift to more psychotic-like states as part of an organized defence system which may well be maladaptive but is also effective in quashing pananxiety (1974: 352). Kernberg amplified this view by noting that 'shifting ego states correspond to organized self- and object-representations which are activated for defensive purposes, for primary and secondary gains, to deal with frustration and anxiety' (1983a: 115).

Winnicott (1967a) agreed that a personalized defence organization could be seen in borderline, schizoid and psychotic children which, like Bettelheim's idea of a fortress, acts as a protection that offers invulnerability. Panic itself, according to Winnicott, can be 'an organised awfulness arranged around a phobic situation whose aim [in the defence organization] is to protect the individual from new examples of the unpredictable' (1967a: 199).

In defining the defensive set-up of the borderline child from a Contemporary Freudian perspective, Fonagy (1991; 1995) uses terms like 'defensive inhibition' and 'defensive disavowal' to underscore the active way in which deficit operates within the child's defensive system. He vividly described how a bereaved 5-year-old girl could not bear the idea of the analyst representing her lost father; she could readily accept the analyst as a real person, and could just as easily pretend (in play) that the analyst was the father, but it was too painful to accept the analyst as *representing* the father, because this would necessitate recognizing an object lost. For the time being, the child had recruited a deficit into her defensive system to forestall certain aspects of her mourning process (Fonagy 1995a). The use of Freud's term 'disavowal' is particularly apt in indicating the *partial* impairments of borderline functioning – developmentally some cognitive capacities are present, but they become narrowed for defensive purposes.

When primitive defences that are 'normal' fail for the child, Kleinian writers have stressed the use of defensive organizations as stabilizers, against both paranoid states (Joseph 1981) and the pain of depressive states (Steiner 1979). The defences may be primitive but their arrangement is usually sophisticated in order to screen out unbearable mental states and to keep developmental challenges in a narrow band. Indeed, these organizations may be the means by which 'states' become 'traits'. Jackson (1985), reporting from a Kleinian perspective, described how a pre-adolescent borderline boy employed pseudo-congeniality, a mechanical use of words, and a sudden withdrawal into empty-mindedness as building blocks for a defensive system against emotional contact and growth.

Regression or developmental arrest?

When early American contributors like Geleerd (1946), Weil (1953a) and Mahler *et al.* (1949) described their patients as 'pre-psychotic' or 'insidiously psychotic', they based their formulations on the observation that portions of the ego had developed and become organized up to a certain point. This made it logical for them to explain the child's pathology in terms of 'developmental arrest' or 'inadequate progression', though the presence of some ego development also led these authors to refer to regressive levels of organization. Subsequent writers like Pine (1974), Masterson (1972) and Kernberg (1983a), reaching up to today's contributors like Alvarez (1992), Bleiberg (1994) and Cohen *et al.* (1994), have all framed their aetiologic formulations within a developmental failure model – validated in many instances by successful analytic interventions where delays and deficits have been shown to be reversible.

Anna Freud did not believe that regression to a symbiotic phase alone could explain borderline disturbance, which she preferred to conceptualize in terms of a *fundamental* defect in the child's capacity to maintain an object cathexis (Rosenfeld and Sprince 1963: 619). This defect is therefore primarily libidinal and reflects an extreme disparity between the level of maturity of the ego and superego and the level of drive activity. The result is a serious hold-up in development. Contemporary writers, though, are apt to think of a more active process when referring to inhibition than is embodied in the notion of delay or arrest. Fonagy (1991), for example, suggests that borderline pathology is defined by an inhibition of mental functions and processes, culminating in a non-awareness of mental states in the self and others. He also considers the possibility that some deficits are self-imposed – as part of a 'defensive disavowal'. This touches on the theme of defensive organizations mentioned above.

For Klein (1930a; 1932) the concept of inhibition was always favoured over regression because in practice she had encountered many instances of how mental capacities in the child, including a stable object cathexis, had come to a standstill as a result of the developing ego's failure to master sadism, only to see capacities reactivated through clinical intervention. Of a 9-year-old psychotic boy who barely spoke, who had never drawn a picture, and who stopped playing at 4 but who began to respond in treatment, she said, 'What appeared now, therefore, were sublimations rescued from profound repression, partly in the form of revivals, and partly as new creations' (1932: 70).

Borderline *psychotic*?

Should we not simply regard these children as psychotic, as Pine (1974) suggests? There is certainly strong agreement among authors that what keenly distinguishes this group of children symptomatically is their leaning towards a psychotic constellation. Geleerd (1946) referred to these children as 'pre-psychotic'. Ekstein and Wallerstein (1954) claimed that, while mature ways of relating exist in these children, the 'dominant cast' of their relationships is autistic/symbiotic. This is in line with Mahler *et al.*'s (1949) concept of a continuum from 'benign' to 'malignant' forms of childhood psychosis, based on Mahler's own use of the concept of infantile psychosis. Following *DSM-III-R* proscriptions, Pine (1974) excluded infantile autism or symbiotic psychosis from the symptomatic domain of borderline children – otherwise he saw no real distinction between this and other forms of psychosis in childhood. In Kleinian psychology a continuum concept from neurotic to psychotic is certainly implicit in the notion of infantile psychosis, which can be manifest across different developmental levels depending on the extremity and coincidence of internal and external factors (Isaacs 1943; Hughes 1988).

Essentially this touches upon the question of which 'border' we are considering when assessing the 'in-betweenness' of borderline pathology – the psychotic border? the neurotic border? In addition, are we speaking of micro-psychotic symptoms that clear up, or are we referring to an underlying psychotic core that is continuously vulnerable to stress? To some degree these are questions and concerns borrowed from debates in the adult literature; for children perhaps the more important question to ask is – for what reasons in today's context do we require specificity in making this diagnosis? To judge by the focus of so much of the current literature, it seems tempting to suggest that specificity is needed around the overlap with Axis I disorders like Conduct Disorder, Attention Deficit and Hyperactivity Disorder and Separation Anxiety Disorder. But I believe this would be looking in the wrong direction. With the organic border ruled out for borderlines, and with the neurotic categories pretty well annotated, the answer must surely lie in another direction – we need to be more precise about *which* psychotic symptoms are pathogenomic of this group. This remains the key issue relating to specificity, in my view, if the term 'borderline' is to have any contemporary diagnostic relevance (see Conclusion, pp. 35–8).

While it is true that child clinicians vary as to which border they consider paramount, and therefore about whether psychotic features are first- or second-rank symptoms, they nevertheless agree about the significance of psychotic functioning in the area of ego organization and object relations (Pine 1983). Freud's (1937) comment that every normal person's ego approximates to that of the psychotic to a greater or lesser degree implies a continuity of psychotic and non-psychotic aspects of the mind in all individuals, an idea that deviates significantly from the requirements of a formal psychiatric model which requires a clear perimeter between psychotic and non-psychotic phenomena (Tarnopolsky *et al.* 1995). However, the notion of continuity, or indeed of the coexistence of normality and pathology, seems to be particularly appropriate for children, whose development is still in progress, whose approach to reality testing is irreducible to adult forms, and for whom normal and abnormal incursions on ego functions are a typical feature of development. Within psychoanalytic definitions, therefore, the idea of incursions from a psychotic 'twin' upon the normal part of the personality, which inhibits mental representations or interferes with normal mental functioning, may provide a common-sense theoretical view of the fluctuating ego organization and object relations so often encountered in borderline children (Bion 1957).

Therapeutic goals and techniques

Work with this borderline group of children, where the internal picture may be so chaotic as to challenge our conceptions of what passes in the psyche as structure, presents the clinician with special challenges. These challenges have highlighted, as a source of solidarity, the fact that, whatever their theoretical background, therapists are facing common clinical problems. The special peculiarities of uneven drive, ego and superego development have also meant that, in order to accommodate these children in treatment, the different schools within child analysis have undertaken some adjustments to their respective techniques. These adjustments, fittingly, have brought them closer together in conceptual thinking as well. On one point, though, everyone is in agreement – the therapist will be more active than usual as an agent of psychic change.

In Kleinian technique these changes have been tied up with a reappraisal of the developmental constituents of the paranoid-schizoid position. Alvarez (1985; 1992) distinguished between defences against psychic pain and defences that are gropings towards structure and agency. In her work she found that what is critical is being able to discern when classic borderline defences like splitting, idealization, projective identification are ego-limiting or ego-enhancing. Technically this requires the installation of 'advanced listening posts' to discern variations in the form of the child's material. 'The content may be the same but the change in form may signal the beginnings of a capacity for symbolisation' (1985: 99). In a similar vein, the content of the therapist's interpretations may need to be more 'diplomatic' – the use of *mental* language over part-object language is recommended. The goal of these technical modifications is to make room for the awakening or reclamation of psychic functions (Alvarez 1992: Ch. 4). While part-object language may pose problems, especially where primary-process thinking is prevalent, my own view is that the standard technique developed by Kleinian therapists of always striving to phrase interpretations around the most prominent *anxiety* of the moment contains an inbuilt 'diplomatic' component with respect to the child's listening level.

Several different approaches emerged in the USA – all within a multi-modal paradigm. Geleerd (1946) adopted a method which combined analysis with peripatetic support which she claimed maximized the transference relationship. Weil (1973) recommended a preliminary phase of educational support as a prelude to analytic work. Sherick et al. (1978) suggested a measure of ego support in parallel to interpretative work based on an ongoing assessment of the ego. Support of, and intervention in, the child's outside world was also recommended by Kernberg (1983b), but this was effected in conjunction with analytic work which technically focuses on interpretations of 'live' transference themes inside the sessions (e.g. evidence of twinship or rapprochement-type transferences). The importance of 'here-and-now' interventions that actively verbalize and address fantasy distortions are stressed in the service of promoting secondary-process thinking. Pine (1976) also agreed that psychoanalytic therapy, as it is conventionally applied, can be successful in treating borderline disturbance, but an awareness of current developmental attainments and the specific form of the pathology should guide the clinician in his or her choice of technique.

Geleerd (1946) worked within the residential school setting at the Menninger Clinic, and therefore emphasized the importance of school as a powerful therapeutic milieu, especially in respect to the demand for reality principle functioning. Weil recommended analytic support via supervision for teachers who discover border-line children in their classrooms. Later US authors like Schimmer (1983) were to confirm the prognostic value of this combination of school and therapy – which has also found support among therapists working in UK schools (Jackson 1970; Woods 1985; Lubbe 1986).

The problem of what to interpret, and whether interpretations should be content- or support-directed, has highlighted areas of divergence among different theoretical approaches. Of special concern has been the use of 'trigger language', i.e. words that might precipitate acting out or a regression to a symbiotic trans-ference (Ekstein and Wallerstein 1957). Such a concern was also echoed by Rosenfeld and Sprince (1965), who drew attention to the technical plight of the therapist working verbally with children who are dominated by primary-process thinking. As an antidote to problems of signal words, Ekstein and Wallerstein (1957) explored the use of what they termed 'symbolic acts' – play actions where the therapist consciously enters into a role which can be embroidered upon in the interests of investigating sensitive subjects or feelings.

Alvarez (1985; 1989) examined some of these debates around what constitutes an interpretation in child work and noted that the more disturbed the child the broader the concept of interpretation needs to be. All therapists, she argued, practise some degree of tact and self-regulation with respect to the developmental level of the patient's functioning, and they modify their interpretations accordingly to accommodate what the patient has not yet owned – especially in latency cases and in cases where the therapist is required to address both sides of the border between sanity and madness (1989: 81).

At the Anna Freud Centre 'developmental psychotherapy' is how contemporary workers describe their approach to children with 'mixed psychopathology' (Fonagy and Target 1996a; Fonagy et al. in press). This approach is based on a psychopathology model that depicts borderline disturbance as an inhibition or disengagement of a whole cluster of mental representations and processes, resulting in a variety of developmental deficits. A flexible combination of techniques is employed to liberate these inhibitions and to restore to the child its mental capacities, pre-eminently the child's capacity for self- and object-representations. These techniques involve performing certain functions which the child is as yet incapable of. They include:

(i) encouraging distinctions between reality and fantasy, thought and action, cause and effect through verbalization by the therapist as a benign real object;
(ii) focusing on communication and thinking capacity (this can be done through providing a verbal commentary on events that are taking place and can include the therapist's own thoughts about curious and puzzling happenings – this brings about an awareness that the object has a mental life);
(iii) encouraging, through example, the labelling of emotions to promote affect regulation and impulse control. Such 'partial' interpretations can be expanded into transference interpretations when self- and object-representations are more differentiated;
(iv) object-relations support through direct action by the therapist, like practising social skills or using role play to help with separations – the goal being not merely to impart a skill but to facilitate ego functions that underlie learning.

All these strategies, and others not mentioned here, are directed at deficits in *mental functioning* and the interpersonal ramifications of these deficits. In this respect object-relations schools in the UK are nowadays much closer in their clinical theories, i.e. in their conception of pathology and their therapy goals and strategies. A focus on the developmental acquisition of mental processes, their origins in the caregiving environment, the impact of the curtailment of mental processes upon object relations and symbolic communication, and the concept of therapeutic action as the 'reactivation' or 'reclamation' of inhibited mental functions, are themes around which the traditions of Kleinian, Winnicottian and Contemporary Freudian therapists have found increasing convergence.

Interpersonal use of the therapist

All the prominent reviews and overviews have stressed disturbed interpersonal relationships as a core symptom category in borderline children (Vela *et al.* 1983; Goldman *et al.* 1992; Bleiberg 1994). In therapy, these disturbances quickly establish themselves as a feature of the transference, and they tend to get expressed through action communications and other pre-linguistic forms of communication which find their way into the interaction between child and therapist.

One particular type of interaction has been frequently described by therapists working within different theoretical systems, namely, the excessive unconscious use of the therapist as a symbiotic partner for the purposes of self-cohesion. The therapist becomes a 'container' for the child's need to centre himself or herself emotionally, and this typically involves manoeuvring the therapist into a particular role (or the unwitting enactment thereof) as a substitute for the experience of intolerable feelings that cannot yet be encompassed within the child's mind – a form of actualization of the transference. Anna Freud (1965) refers to this role in terms of an auxiliary ego function, which in borderline cases acts to strengthen the patient's sanity. So common is this feature of the work with borderline children that many authors regard its presence as diagnostic.

In the USA Chethik and Fast (1970) were the first to draw attention to the interpersonal use of the therapist by the child for the purposes of fulfilling a particular fantasy – which can have a defensive as well as developmental motive. Referring to the enactment of omnipotent fantasies, Bleiberg (1994) also mentions the child's 'rigid and desperate insistence on inducing interpersonal responses that support an illusory perspective' which can put the therapist under enormous strain and present a stern test for the concept of analytic neutrality.

Kleinian therapists have traditionally regarded these manoeuvres as based on pathological projective identification, an omnipotent defence with an interpersonal dimension that interferes with the capacity for verbal and abstract thinking, culminating in a concretization of the mental processes and causing a confusion between reality and phantasy (Rosenfeld 1987). When the therapist is used in this way as a representative of the child's ego, Alvarez (1985; 1992) regards it as an *adaptive* feature of projective identification, as opposed to its purely defensive function. In a similar vein Fonagy (1991) declares that because developmental failure to 'mentalize' feelings and thoughts is such a prominent feature in the clinical picture, in therapy it is essential that children be given opportunities for discovering their minds in the existence of the other. Chused (1995) also emphasizes the developmental aspect of enactments by showing that when the therapist is a partial or a non-active participant in such enactments they can be mutative by virtue of disconfirming transference expectations.

Conclusion

Once we decide to disregard the diagnostic categories derived from descriptive psychiatry for adult psychopathology and to play down the importance of symptomology as such, we can hope to be alerted more vigorously to ... other aspects of patient's personality. Where children are concerned, these will be mostly developmental ones.

(Anna Freud 1956: 307)

This chapter has sought to keep the focus on *children*. Far too frequently in reviews and discussions of borderline pathology, child versions of the diagnosis have been intermingled with their adult counterparts, in matters of history, theory, aetiology, psychodynamics, symptom clusters, etc. Historically, it has been claimed that developments in child diagnosis tend to shadow those in adult nomenclatures (Shapiro 1983), but one of the purposes of this chapter is to show that the borderline concept as applied to children has its own origins and lines of development that start with work with psychotic children. While in some respects this mirrors the history of the adult diagnosis, it is important to free the childhood version from some of the theoretical wrangles, research contests and political lobbies that have sprung up around the massive interest in the adult disorder. This has led, I believe, to a number of distortions of key issues relating to theory and clinical methods of working with children – like the role of maturational factors and the debate about whether personality disorders exist in children.

The Psychoanalytic Glossary (Moore and Fine 1968) defines 'borderline' as referring to 'conditions which manifest both neurotic and psychotic phenomena without fitting unequivocally into either diagnostic category' (1968: 24). Clearly this definition, which is very close to the one used by the pioneers in child work, does not suggest that a borderline disorder in childhood occurs on

an indeterminate border. Nor does it suggest that borderline symptoms cut across a variety of other disorders, or that a patchwork
diagnosis is necessary for this group of children. What it states is
that such children are not autistic or schizophrenic or any subtype
of these, and that their problems, which may appear severely
neurotic, cannot be entirely understood within the framework of
infantile neurosis. It is not that they don't fit in anywhere, it is
that traditional categories don't quite accommodate them because
they comprise a special group occupying a region between
neurosis and psychosis owing to specific developmental imbalances. Clearly, the analytic setting was the ideal setting for these
'in-between' disturbances to be uncovered for the first time.
Furthermore, the fact that their problems can be framed using
developmental principles does not mean that evidence of their
psychotic functioning should be regarded as 'secondary' or viewed
as being 'soft' in nature.

Of course, as many authors have found (Frijling-Schreuder
1969; Pine 1974; Chethik 1980), the hazard of defining a *distinct*
borderline category for children has been in settling upon the
correct criteria for distinguishing this diagnosis from those made
under neurotic and psychotic categories – and in particular at the
margins of these categories. In applying the term, child clinicians
have shadowed their adult colleagues in being governed by traditional diagnostic conceptions of what is psychotic and what is
non-psychotic – the two being clearly demarcated. Hence, they
have tended to lean in one direction or another when defining the
disorder, even when using dynamic principles. That is, they have
approached the diagnosis either from the vertex of defective
neurotic structure or from the perspective of an underlying
psychotic core. Among psychoanalytic child practitioners this has
been played out along the lines of different theoretical predilec-
tions: between those clinicians working from the concept of the
infantile neurosis (and beyond) and those whose work is under-
pinned by the concept of infantile psychosis.

The pioneers, of course, placed these children on the psychotic
or near-psychotic border, but the main problem in recent times
has been a loss of specificity of the concept in the face of several
developments in contemporary practice. Bleiberg (1994) has noted,
for example, that nowadays Axis I disorders like conduct disorders, Attention Deficit Disorder, eating disorders, mood disorders
and Post-traumatic Stress Disorder appear frequently in the

diagnosis of borderline youngsters. The danger here, as Kernberg and Shapiro (1990) points out, is that co-morbidity can be used to obscure the presence of psychotic features, a pitfall that Melanie Klein (1930b) drew attention to a long time ago. My own impression is that many children who previously attracted a borderline psychotic diagnosis nowadays receive a diagnosis of Asperger's syndrome as a means of sanctioning *some* psychotic signs. How could this loss of specificity be addressed?

It has been suggested that in adults the inclusion of psychotic symptoms in the diagnosis of Borderline Personality Disorder decreases the specificity of the diagnosis (Widiger *et al.* 1992), though this has now been partially implemented in the *DSM-IV*. While this may be true for adults, especially those with mood disorders, in children I believe the opposite would hold true. The inclusion of psychotic symptoms would increase specificity for the following reasons.

(i)   It would ensure that developmental considerations of arrest and deviation would gain ascendancy over regression hypotheses normally associated with adult borderline disturbance, and with other developmental disorders in childhood of a pervasive form.

(ii) Making psychotic features a requirement would also compel clinicians to specify those features that are diagnostic of borderline disturbance and those that are diagnostic of schizotypal disorder, not only in the realm of cognitive distortions but also in the realm of object relations deficits.

(iii) The special type of anxiety that many authors regard as pathogenomic in these children can correctly be termed 'psychotic anxiety', and differentiated from other forms of anxiety that are expressed in a manifest form only.

(iv) Including psychotic symptoms would permit a borderline diagnosis to be made before the age of 6 – a common feature of the work undertaken by early contributors.

(v)   Accordingly, treatment techniques and objectives would become better focused towards these specific features, and their developmental component would be formally recognized.

The inclusion of psychotic symptoms would therefore make the diagnosis more restrictive but more clinically proficient, I believe. Hence the preference given to the term 'borderline psychotic' in the title of this book.

Clinicians are often reluctant, even today, to make a diagnosis of psychosis in childhood. Dickes (1974) commented that many workers seem to regard this diagnosis as a form of name-calling. It is frequently claimed that children showing borderline disturbance carry symptoms that cut across a variety of classifiable disorders. Doubtless these claims are intended to reflect the diagnostic puzzle presented by these children, but they also serve to underplay psychotic features by letting them recede into the background of the clinical picture. Similarly, defining borderline disturbance in very general terms as a developmental disorder or as a personality disorder can also serve to 'tone down' the presence of psychotic phenomena, which are then relegated to the status of 'associated features'. The result, I believe, is an underdiagnosis of psychotic symptoms in a group of children whose problems, when they were highlighted for the first time, were found to include both neurotic and psychotic signs.

Chapter 2

Borderline Personality Disorder in children and adolescents

Efrain Bleiberg

In 1983 Pine reported that, in clinical practice, the flow of children who were given the diagnosis 'borderline' had reached flood proportions. Twenty-five years later the 'flood' has not receded, yet the concept of borderline disorders or borderline personality in children and adolescents remains mired in unclarity and controversy.

Striving for an empirical, atheoretical classification, successive editions of the *Diagnostic and Statistical Manual of Mental Disorders* or *DSM* (American Psychiatric Association (APA) 1980; 1987; 1994) designated borderline as a specific personality disorder – the Borderline Personality Disorder (BPD) – which in *DSM*, 4th edition (*DSM-IV*, APA 1994), is included in one of three clusters of personality disorders. This cluster – the cluster B or the 'dramatic' personality disorders – also includes the Histrionic, the Narcissistic and the Antisocial Personality Disorders. According to *DSM-IV* (APA 1994), BPD consists of 'a pervasive pattern of instability of interpersonal relationships, self-image, affects, and control over impulses, *beginning by early adulthood* [emphasis added]' (1994: T: 5), a definition which, age of onset aside, echoes Ekstein and Wallerstein's idea of 'stable instability'.

DSM-IV's approach to BPD, however, raises several questions about the applicability of this diagnosis in childhood and adolescence: are there enough empirical data to support the notion of BPD as a distinct diagnostic entity in childhood? More generally, is it valid to ascertain the diagnosis of 'personality disorder' in children or adolescents? Personality disorders, after all, are defined as relatively enduring and pervasively maladaptive patterns of experiencing, coping and relating. Yet children and adolescents are engaged in fluid developmental processes in which every aspect of their bodies and personalities is constantly changing, at different rates, creating new equilibria and disequilibria within them and in their relationships with their environment. Maturation and experience provide children with ever-changing tools to cope with, perceive and organize their experience, as well as to relate to others, making it difficult, if not impossible, to speak of 'rigid and enduring patterns'.

Even if personality disorders could be diagnosed before adulthood, are there developmental and clinical continuities between borderline children, borderline adolescents and borderline adults? Does 'borderline' refer to a primitive level of personality development or is it instead a specific disorder, as *DSM-IV* advocates? Or should borderline be considered a dimensional diagnosis, extending from less severe forms – such as the identity disorders – to more severe presentations? Or is borderline part of a cluster that includes other personality disorders with common clinical, developmental or aetiological features? Last, but not least, what are the links between BPD in children and adolescents and other common Axis I diagnoses such as Conduct Disorder, Substance Abuse, Separation Anxiety Disorder, Mood Disorder, Attention-Deficit Disorder, Eating Disorder, Dissociative Disorder, Somatoform Disorder, and Post-traumatic Stress Disorder? The high prevalence of these Axis I diagnoses in various combinations in BPD youngsters raises the question of whether 'borderline' is a designation for atypical, complicated, or severe forms of Axis I diagnosis. In particular, the very common finding of a history of protracted trauma – physical abuse and neglect and, very significantly, sexual abuse – in borderline adolescents and adults raises the question (Goodwin *et al.* 1990; Herman 1992) of whether 'borderline' is little more than a pejorative designation for individuals who suffer a complex PTSD syndrome as a consequence of chronic abuse and victimization.

These questions are far from settled. This chapter will review (1) clinical features of BPD in children and adolescents; (2) current ideas about the role of psychodynamic, developmental, neurobiological, family interaction and traumatic factions in the aetiology and pathogenesis of BPD; (3) a proposed model to conceptualize the development of personality disorders and BPD, in children and adolescents, and (4) a treatment approach based on such model.

Clinical features of BPD in children and adolescents

In spite of conceptual disagreements, Bemporad *et al.* (1982) and Vela *et al.* (1983) found substantial consensus in the clinical literature regarding diagnostic criteria for borderline children. Bemporad *et al.* (1982) outlined the following diagnostic features: (1) a paradigmatic fluctuation of functioning, with rapid shifts between psychotic-like and neurotic levels of reality testing; (2) a lack of 'signal anxiety' (Freud 1926) and a proneness to states of panic dominated by overwhelming concerns of body dissolution, annihilation, or abandonment; (3) a disruption in thought processes and content that shifts rapidly into loose, idiosyncratic thinking; (4) an impairment in relationships and, when under stress, great difficulty in distinguishing self from others, in appreciating other people's needs and point of view, or in integrating disparate emotional experiences about self and others; and (5) a lack of impulse control, including an inability to contain intense affects, delay gratification, control rage, or modulate destructive and self-destructive tendencies. Along similar lines, Vela *et al.* (1983) described the following features: (1) disturbances in interpersonal relationships; (2) disturbances in the sense of reality; (3) excessive anxiety; (4) severe impulse problems; (5) 'neurotic-like' symptoms; and (6) uneven or distorted development.

Upon closer scrutiny, however, it has become increasingly apparent that children described in the literature as borderline seem to fall into two rather distinct groups (Petti and Vela 1990). Both groups present significant disturbance of social and emotional development, including marked impairment of peer relationships, affect regulation, frustration tolerance and impulse control, as well as poor self-esteem and poor self-image. Children in one group, however, show a more fragile reality contact and thought organization. Idiosyncratic, magical thinking pervades their lives, acquiring greater intensity in emotionally charged contexts or when they are faced with lack of structure. Shy and friendless, they retreat to a world of fantasy, haunted by ideas of reference, by suspiciousness, and by discomfort in social situations. Their ability to make sense of human exchanges and empathize with others is strikingly limited. They are impoverished in their capacity to communicate, which is further hampered by the oddness of their speech and the constriction or inappropriateness of their affect.

These children, as Petti and Vela (1990) report, have a greater chance of a family history of a schizophrenia-spectrum disorder. More likely, these youngsters are *not* in a development continuum with adolescents or adults with BPD, although longitudinal studies are needed to test out this premise. Descriptively, they resemble a range of *DSM-IV* diagnoses that include schizotypal and schizoid personality disorder which *DSM-IV* groups in the Cluster A or the 'odd' personality disorder, as well as with milder forms of pervasive developmental disorders and the children Cohen *et al.* (1994) described as multicomplex developmental disorders. Characterizing these 'odd' children as borderline has fostered diagnostic unclarity. Such unclarity has been resolved in the studies of adults with BPD which have differentiated BPD – and related 'dramatic' personality disorders such as Histrionic, Narcissistic and Antisocial Personality Disorders – from the 'odd' and the 'anxious' clusters of personality disorders (Gunderson 1984). Furthermore, empirical studies have also put to rest the notion that BPD was a schizophrenia-spectrum disorder (Wender 1977; Stone 1979).

By contrast, a second group of children present features more closely resembling those found in the Cluster B or the 'Dramatic' Personality Disorder, including intense, dramatic affect and hunger for social response – but not odd thinking and communication or avoidance of social contact. These children are clingy and vulnerable to separation and prone to hyperactivity and temper tantrums. In early development they often present 'disorganized' patterns of attachment – erratic, unpredictable alternations of approach, avoidance and 'trance-like' behaviour in the presence of caregivers. Their history often reveals 'difficult' temperament, that is, a pattern of high activity level, poor adaptability, negative mood and problems settling into rhythmic patterns of sleep, wakefulness and feeding. Cranky and hard to soothe, these infants frequently challenge and burden their caregivers. This chapter addresses this second group of youngsters.

By school age, borderline children almost invariably meet diagnostic criteria for an Axis I diagnosis, more commonly Attention-Deficit Hyperactivity Disorder, Conduct Disorder, Separation Anxiety Disorder, or Mood Disorder. Many of these youngsters appear anxious, moody, irritable and explosive. Minor upsets or frustrations trigger intense affective storms, episodes of uncontrolled emotion wholly out of proportion to the apparent precipitant. These affective storms mirror the kaleidoscopic quality of these children's experience of self and others. One moment they feel elated and blissfully connected in perfect love and harmony with an idealized partner. But at the next moment, they plunge into bitter disappointment and rage, coupled with self-loathing and despair.

Self-centredness is a striking characteristic of these children. They need constant attention and respond with rage to rejection or indifference. Alternating between idealization and devaluation, they seductively and manipulatively strive to coerce others into providing them with a stream of emotional supplies.

On clinical examination, borderline school-age children may appear helpless and vulnerable, provocative and suspicious, or eager to comply and ingratiate themselves with the examiner. Leichtman and Nathan (1983) described how these youngsters quickly attempt to establish controlling relationships with the examiner. Some show surprisingly little anxiety about meeting alone with the clinician and proceed to take over the office as if they owned it. But even those who seem vulnerable and anxious try vigorously to set the agenda for the meeting. They become anxious and even more desperate and arbitrary when the examiner does not meet their demands or when they feel that their control is threatened.

Indeed, these children direct much of their energy at coercing others into assuming particular roles. As Chethik and Fast (1970) pointed out, they demand that others become players in a vivid fantasy world of their own creation. It is in the enactment of these fantasies with others that they seem to come to life.

The developmental and psychosocial pressures of adolescence typically trigger the onset of the full range of borderline symptomatology, allowing for greater diagnostic certainty. Unstable relationships become prominent as transient idealization and clingy overdependence alternate with rage, devaluation and feelings of abandonment and betrayal. Promiscuity and self-mutilation are more common in borderline girls, whereas aggression, coupled with hidden fears of rejection, is more typical of boys. Drugs, alcohol, or food binges become common strategies to block feelings of subjective dyscontrol, fragmentation and loneliness, often brought about by disruptions in relationships such as separations or failure to find the 'right' balance between closeness and distance. Yet while food, drugs or sex can bring transient comfort they typically lead only to shame, guilt and dreaded feelings of inner deadness. Suicidal and parasuicidal behaviours come to the fore in an effort to release tension or restore the capacity to feel alive; as attempts to escape anxiety and depression; as punishment to disappointing or abandoning partners; or as manoeuvres to evoke guilt and involvement from others.

Aetiology and pathogenesis

Psychodynamic and developmental theories

A range of related hypotheses have emerged from the psychoanalytic literature to explain the aetiology of borderline personality and BPD in children and adolescents. Mahler's (1971; Mahler *et al.* 1975) ideas about the separation–individuation process and Otto Kernberg's (1967; 1975) notions about splitting have provided the most influential conceptual framework for psychodynamic clinicians in the USA.

According to Mahler, children between 12 and 36 months of age go through a series of stages during which: (1) they internalize some of the soothing, equilibrium-maintaining functions previously performed exclusively by the parents, thus acquiring the capacity to carry out these functions with some degree of autonomy; (2) they practise ego skills and use them to expand their knowledge of themselves and the world and to figure out how to evoke desired responses from the environment; and (3) they integrate the 'good' and the 'bad' representations of the self and the object. These achievements, in turn, permit children to accept the reality of their existence as separate individuals and to develop object constancy, which refers to the ability to maintain relationships and evoke the loving and comforting image of the object in spite of separation or frustration.

Both Mahler and Kernberg believe that derailment of this developmental process results in borderline psychopathology. For Kernberg, the basic pathogenic factor is excessive aggression, whether derived from a constitutional propensity or secondary to undue early frustration, which leads to a predominance of negative introjects. The child's aggressive introjects threaten to destroy the 'good' images of the self and the object, fostering the defensive need to maintain a split of the good and bad representations. The central feature of borderline pathology, according to Kernberg, is the ongoing effort to hold on to an 'all-good' or idealized image of the self and the object in the face of unremitting assault from 'all-bad' introjects, activated by separation, frustration, or the object's failure to live up to ideal expectations.

Masterson and Rinsley (1975) claimed that specific patterns of mother–infant interaction thwart the separation–individuation process and lead to borderline psychopathology. In their view, the mothers of future borderline individuals take pride in and find gratification in their children's dependency. These mothers reward passive-dependent, clinging behaviour while withdrawing from or otherwise punishing their children for actively striving for autonomy. They carefully attune to states of helplessness and proximity-seeking behaviour but give subtle or overt rebuffs when their children show evidence of mastery or independence. The central message communicated to these children, said Rinsley (1984), is that to grow up is to face 'the loss or withdrawal of material supplies, coupled with the related injunction that to avoid that calamity the child must remain dependent, inadequate, symbiotic' (1984: 5).

Such selectivity of maternal response and attunement fosters a split of the maternal representation into two components: one rewarding and gratifying in response to dependency, and the second punitive and withdrawing in response to autonomy, mastery and separation. This representational split and the associated inhibition of autonomy come to the fore at times when developmental and psychosocial pressures push towards separation, particularly during adolescence.

Adler (1985) postulated that the central feature of borderline psychopathology is the patient's inability to evoke the memory of a soothing, comforting object when facing separation or distress. Adler attributed this defect in internalization to parental failure in providing an adequate 'holding environment', as described by Winnicott (1965). The consequence is an inner sense of emptiness; reliance on transitional objects and activities, similar to the early transitional experiences described by Winnicott (1953), such as drugs or food to provide soothing and comfort; and angry, manipulative efforts to produce involvement and attention from others.

Gabbard (1994) cogently summarized the controversies and critiques surrounding the psychodynamic models of BPD. He pointed out the overemphasis in most psychodynamic models on early development, particularly the separation–individuation process, at the expense of other, also sensitive developmental

stages, such as the Oedipal phase and adolescence. Equally significant is the lack of consideration of constitutional factors – except
for Otto Kernberg, who has been criticized for ascribing *too much*
significance to constitutionally based aggression. Constitutional
vulnerability plays a major role in shaping the child's developing
intrapsychic world by affecting the negotiation of developmental
tasks and by influencing parental responses – which in turn influence the child's experience. Psychodynamic hypotheses also tend
to exaggerate maternal responsibility and largely ignore the role
of others – particularly neglectful and/or abusive fathers – in the
pathogenesis of BPD.

Biological theories

For the past 15 years, a growing consensus has emerged regarding
the significance of biological factors in the aetiology of Borderline
Personality Disorder. Specific biological vulnerabilities both shape
the intrapsychic development of children with BPD and evoke the
interpersonal responses that maintain, reinforce, or exacerbate
the intrapsychic configuration of these children. Much higher rates
of parental psychopathology have been identified in children with
the diagnosis of BPD (Goldman *et al.* 1993). Goldman *et al.*'s
findings parallel the reports of higher rates of depressive disorders, antisocial personality and substance abuse disorders in the
families of adults with BPD. Although these reports suggest a
biological diathesis, spelling out the nature of this vulnerability
remains controversial.

  Klein (1977) first proposed that at least a subgroup of borderline patients, whom he referred to as 'hysteroid dysphorics', suffer
from a problem in affective regulation that gives rise to emotional
lability and heightened sensitivity to rejection. According to Klein,
manipulative relationships and other maladaptive interpersonal
tactics and object relations are the result and not the cause of
affective dysregulation. This view gained strength after the studies
of Stone (1979), Stone *et al.* (1981) and Akiskal (1981). Stone
found a high prevalence of affective disorder in the relatives of
borderline patients, but no increase in schizophrenia-spectrum
disorders. Akiskal identified features suggestive of borderline
personality disorder in the offspring of affectively ill patients, and
proposed that these patients may represent an atypical or incip-
ient form of affective disorder.

These studies helped to distinguish borderline personality disorder from schizophrenia and suggested instead a connection with the mood disorders. More recent studies, summarized by Gunderson and Zanarini (1989), have confirmed an elevated prevalence of mood disorders in the relatives of borderline probands, but have also pointed out that a linkage between borderline personality and mood disorders is neither uniform nor strong. Yet, for a significant number of borderline children, a vulnerability to mood disorders appears greatly to heighten their chances for major disruptions in personality development and strongly to predispose these children to develop BPD.

Case example

Travis illustrates the plight of these children. His birth was haunted by the suicides of his father, a paternal uncle and a paternal grandfather, all suffering from bipolar disorder. Travis's father, also named Travis, had pleaded with his wife to have an abortion. When she refused, he hanged himself – three months before Travis's birth. Travis later was told that his father had 'gotten so excited when he found out that Travis was coming' that his blood pressure went 'sky high' and he died of a heart attack. Not surprisingly, the boy became convinced that he had killed his father.

Mood lability was Travis's most striking clinical feature when he was brought for consultation at the age of 7. One moment, he bubbled with enthusiasm, swept up by an elated mood while his thoughts raced ebulliently. Yet minor mistakes or frustrations triggered fits of rage or led him to plunge into abject ignominy and self-hatred. Constant vigilance was needed to prevent him from hurting himself in one or another 'accident'.

A trial of mood-stabilizing medication resulted in a significant decrease in the boy's affective storms. Yet his developmental difficulties remained glaringly apparent. His sense of self and others appeared like an ever-changing kaleidoscope. He valiantly tried to hold on to an image of himself as the heroic saviour and protector of his beautiful mother. This image, however, was constantly besieged by a hateful introject of a guilt-inducing, self-absorbed, depriving mother, with whom he was locked in a rageful embrace.

A proneness to irritability, mood lability and anger seems clearly to interfere with the development of a cohesive sense of self and object constancy. Rage promotes the need to rely on splitting to protect even a semblance of good internal relationships. Just as surely, these frustrating, difficult-to-comfort children burden parents with anger, shame and guilt feelings. Both the parents, who are often vulnerable themselves to mood and personality disorders, and their children end up caught in coercive cycles of hatred and rejection, followed by desperate attempts to re-create blissful reunions.

Other borderline youngsters present a different kind of impulse-control problem. The child psychiatric literature has long emphasized the 'atypical ego development' (Weil 1953a), impulsivity and learning problems of many borderline children. A clinical overlap is readily apparent between the symptoms of the disruptive behaviour disorders – particularly Attention-Deficit Hyperactivity Disorder (ADHD), Conduct Disorder and BPD. Along these lines, Andrulonis et al. (1981) and Andrulonis (1991) have reported on the link between learning disabilities, episodic dyscontrol, or disruptive behaviour disorders in children and BPD in adults.

Impulsive children – and adults – directly translate their wishes, needs and impulses into action, short-circuiting much mediating processing. Because they rush into action, their own wishes cannot evolve into sustained intentions anchored in a sense of stability and self-continuity. In fact, their chronic lack of integration of wishes, needs and motives disrupts their capacity to develop a cohesive and continuous sense of self and others. Their low tolerance of frustration stems from an inability to connect or integrate momentary wishes with general goals and interests, or to form enduring representations of the self and others.

With impulsive youngsters, their actions 'happen' to them instead of resulting from their choice, and thus they experience little sense of guilt or responsibility. The world appears as a disconnected set of temptations and frustrations, possibilities for immediate gain and satisfaction, or obstacles to gratification. They experience other people and relationships in equally fragmentary and shallow ways, which results in an inner life that is barren and undifferentiated.

Marohn et al. (1979) and Offer et al. (1979) have conducted a factor analysis of a sample of juvenile delinquents and concluded that 'borderline' and 'impulsive' constitute two of four overlapping psychological subtypes found in the sample. As Marohn (1991) noted, many of these youngsters have 'little awareness of an inner psychological world, cannot name affects or differentiate one affect from another, and often confuse thought, feeling and deed' (1991: 150). Their concrete, egocentric mode of experience interferes with planning, abstraction and generalization, and forms the basis for their well-known difficulty in learning from experience. Of course, these impulsive, angry youngsters fuel the chaos that often prevails in their families, exhausting their parents and imposing an added burden of frustration and distress while wreaking havoc with what little structure and boundaries their families can offer.

A constitutional proneness to excessive separation anxiety may also play a role in the pathogenesis of BPD in children. Kandel (1983) pointed out a neurobiological readiness to trigger a response of anxiety and hyperarousal in response to the absence of caretakers. The reappearance of caretakers, on the other hand, evokes a 'down regulation' of the alarm system in response to a ready-to-be-activated signal of safety.

Mothers have always known intuitively that infants vary greatly in their 'sturdiness' and overall vulnerability to separations. Primate research (Suomi 1987; 1992) has begun to substantiate such intuition. Baby monkeys vary enormously in their hormonal, autonomic, emotional and behavioural responses to stress, particularly the stress of separation from caretakers. Such variations are also likely in human infants, supporting the contention that separation anxiety disorder has an important constitutional basis.

Children with extreme responses to separation are buffeted by panic and hyperarousal after instances of parental 'abandonment' that would be quite manageable for less vulnerable youngsters. Parental unavailability is utterly devastating for them and promotes clinginess and a desperate need to ensure parental proximity. Parental overinvolvement in these instances may reflect an adaptation to children's fragility rather than an inability to tolerate independence.

As they grow, these anxiously attached (Ainsworth et al. 1978) youngsters carry forward an image of themselves as helpless and incompetent, while they experience others as unavailable, indifferent, or withholding. Rage sometimes turns into disruptive and self-destructive behaviour. Inflicting pain on oneself and causing misery to others can effectively ensure responsiveness from otherwise exhausted or frustrated parents. Thus dramatic behaviour, including outwardly and inwardly directed destructiveness, may become the currency of relatedness every bit as much as it represents a protest against perceived neglect, an unconscious search for confirmation of badness, and an expression of a biologically based predisposition to mischief.

But a straight line cannot be drawn between any of these constitutional vulnerabilities and BPD. Clearly, most children with ADHD, mood disorder, or separation anxiety do *not* become borderline, just as surely as some borderline children appear free of these vulnerabilities. Biological factors can be related to BPD in at least two general ways: (1) developmental association: a major vulnerability, such as ADHD, chronic and present from birth, may greatly increase the likelihood of other problems, burdening families and affecting many spheres of development, thus creating a cascade of negative events that can result in BPD; or (2) ascertainment bias: biological vulnerabilities may multiply the symptoms that disturb others or increase the severity and adjustment difficulties of borderline children, enhancing the chance of bringing borderline children to diagnosis and treatment. Thus clinical surveys of borderline children may overestimate the prevalence of biological factors.

Understanding the pathogenic role of biological factors in BPD also thrusts us into the realm of a transactional perspective: biological factors play an important part in shaping children's experience of themselves and of others; of their competence and of other people's reliability; of the 'safety' or lack of safety of their emotional responses; and of their ability to monitor emotional signals from themselves and from others, to cue others about internal states, and to create states of emotional reciprocity. Biological factors also modify the specific conditions that optimally promote each individual child's development – greater or lesser closeness, limits, structure, and so forth. Last, but not least, biological factors (e.g. irritability, poor adaptability, impulsivity and overactivity) influence parents and shape the parenting that, in turn, shapes children's development – amplifying or minimizing biological vulnerabilities.

Family environment and trauma

As research failed to document a specific constitutional vulnerability or neuropsychiatric dysfunction in the background of individuals with BPD (Van Reeuom *et al.* 1993), the focus of enquiry began to shift to the systematic examination of early family environment – which included an effort to substantiate empirically some of the developmental hypotheses postulated by psychoanalytic clinicians – see section on psychodynamic and developmental theories (pp. 44–6).

Several authors (Frank and Paris 1981; Goldberg *et al.* 1985; Paris and Frank 1989; Paris and Zweig-Frank 1992) have indeed described highly conflictual relationships with mothers, uninvolved fathers, neglectful yet controlling parenting, and chronic discord between the parents. Yet two sets of issues gained prominence as possible pathogenic factors: early loss or separation from the caretakers and physical and sexual abuse.

Parental loss or separation

The fact of the death of a parent is less vulnerable to retrospective distortion. Thus the repeated finding of a history of parental loss during childhood (Stone 1990; Zanarini *et al.* 1989) may be of significance. In a study of adult borderline patients, for example, Stone (1990) identified three subgroups of borderline patients in which approximately 60 per cent had experienced early parental loss: borderline patients who committed suicide, borderline patients with antisocial personality co-morbidity, and schizophreniform-borderline patients.

The impact of a parent's death on children's development has been extensively reviewed in the child psychiatric and psychoanalytic literature (Bleiberg 1991; Furman 1974; Nagera 1970; Wolfenstein 1966).

Although there are significant disagreements about the specific impact of early parental loss and psychopathology, most authors agree that parental loss is, by definition, a significant developmental interference (Nagera 1970). Children require parents to provide psychological regulation and to function as direction-givers, limit-setters, consistent protectors and soothers, interpreters of reality, and facilitators of growth. As Furman (1974) has noted, 'the loss of the vital love object endangers both the building up of the personality and the varied narcissistic satisfactions derived from its functioning' (1974: 53). Interactions with parents form the template in which critical psychological capacities, such as effective self-esteem regulation and object constancy, are forged. Such capacities are essential if children are to achieve meaningful intrapsychic autonomy.

Of course, only a fraction of children who experience the loss of a parent become borderline or develop other forms of psychopathology. This fact supports the conclusion that the pathogenic impact of early parent loss does not depend on the loss alone but is mediated by factors such as gender of child and parent, child's age at the time of the parent's death, quality of the pre-existing relationship, available supports and, particularly, the change the parent's death introduces into the child's family.

A number of studies (e.g. Breier *et al.* 1988; Harris *et al.* 1986) suggest that the chances of subsequent psychopathology are largely determined by the cascade of adverse events precipitated by the death of a parent: protracted depression and unavailability of the surviving parent, financial hardship, disruption of household routines and structure, inconsistent limits, and erratic demands for maturity. In more extreme circumstances, overwhelming stress and social isolation in the surviving parent result in suicidal behaviour; substance abuse; verbal, physical and/or sexual abuse; or parentification of the children (Bleiberg 1991).

Physical and sexual abuse

Physical and especially sexual abuse have emerged in the recent literature as major developmental antecedents of BPD (Goodwin *et al.* 1990; Herman 1992; Herman *et al.* 1989). Indeed, when clinicians open for clinical scrutiny the possibility of sexual abuse, a very large percentage of borderline children and adolescents (Famularo *et al.* 1991; Goldman *et al.* 1992) reveal lives marred by abuse. Theirs is not an empty house, claim Zanarini *et al.* (1989), but a haunted house filled with the terrifying ghosts of caretakers' insensitivity, brutality and boundary violations.

While all traumatic experiences evoke, by definition, a specific psychobiological response that can progress to full-blown PTSD, sexual and physical abuse overwhelm children with special perniciousness. Sexual and physical abuse often involve conditions of protracted, almost inescapable victimization. The perpetrators of sexual and/or physical abuse are commonly the very same people – their caretakers – whom children rely on to help them bring coherence and ascribe meaning to their experience, promote effective coping and adaptive responses, provide relief from stress and tension, and model limit-setting, impulse control and self-regulation. An abundance of research (Pynoos *et al.* 1987; Chu and Dill 1990) demonstrates that children respond more acutely and are less able to overcome the effects of traumatic experiences perpetrated by parents or other family members. Fear of retribution, loyalty conflicts, and concerns about destroying or bringing shame to the entire family militate against disclosure and resolution of these traumatic experiences. Feelings of pleasure and specialness mix in confusing fashion with the pain, rage, shame and helplessness they also feel, compounding their inability to make sense of their plight.

Memories of terrifying, abusive events remain in prolonged, unintegrated storage, prone to activation by traumatic reminders which evoke anew the shock, helplessness, hyperarousal and loneliness of the original trauma (Van der Kolk *et al.* 1997). Not surprisingly, many authors (e.g. Terr 1991) believe that the repeated exposure to physical and/or sexual abuse evokes the distortions in relationship patterns, subjective experience, sense of self, and coping strategies that define the personality disorders. For Terr, 'the defenses and coping mechanisms used in the type II disorders of childhood – long-standing exposure to trauma – massive denial, repression, dissociation, self-anesthesia, self-hypnosis, identification with the aggressor, and aggression turned against the self – often lead to profound character changes' (1991:15–16).

This point requires clarification. Even the highest estimates of sexual abuse in the background of adults with BPD (Herman *et al.* 1989; Ogata *et al.* 1990) are in the range of 60–80 per cent. This suggests that, while sexual abuse is very common in BPD, and indeed is significantly more common in borderline individuals than in controls – in contrast to physical abuse, which is *not* present more significantly in BPD patients than in controls (Paris and Zweig-Frank 1997) – it is nonetheless not *necessary* for the development of BPD. Paris and Zweig-Frank further document that nearly half of a non-borderline sample also reported sexual abuse, supporting the view that sexual abuse is not *sufficient* to develop BPD. Likewise, in Finkelhor and Brown's (1985) sample, 40–70 per cent of individuals with BPD reported sexual abuse compared to 19–26 per cent in a control group – and 25 per cent of the BPD population reported incest compared to 6–12 per cent in the control group, suggesting that the majority of abuse survivors do *not* develop borderline psychopathology. At the same time, sexual abuse, particularly repeated abuse with multiple perpetrators including a parent, and accompanied by threats of physical injury, appears to be associated with borderline psychopathology that includes prominent manifestations of dissociative, or dissociation-related, phenomena such as self-mutilation and other parasuicidal behaviours, depersonalization, derealization and somatoform symptoms (Westen 1990; Chu and Dill 1990).

A large number of studies thus are now converging to support a more complex view of the development of borderline psychopathology that includes the following elements: (a) It is, at best, premature and probably erroneous to consider BPD a chronic post-traumatic disorder. For some borderline patients, as Zanarini and Frankenburg (1997) point out, sexual abuse is not much of an issue, while for others it is an important factor in the development of their maladjustment, and for yet others, it may have been the defining organizer of their lives. (b) Borderline psychopathology results from an admixture of innate vulnerabilities and childhood experiences interacting in various combinations and leading to different subsets of dysfunction that cluster around common features. (c) It is as crucial to understand the significance of constitutional and environmental risk factors as it is to delineate those *protective* factors (both biological and environmental) that allow some children to withstand – without suffering severe maladjustment – environmental assaults and neurobiological misfortune compared to other factors that result in lives of misery and severe psychopathology. The following section presents a model that considers the interaction of protective and risk factors in the development of children with borderline personality.

A proposed model of borderline personality development

A growing body of research (i.e. Beeghly and Cicchetti 1994; Fonagy *et al.* 1994) has begun to examine the interaction of risk and protective factors in generating, organizing, maintaining and reinforcing patterns of adjustment or maladjustment. A key set of questions involves the differences in outcome: What protects *some* children who suffer from biological vulnerabilities and/or early trauma compared to others who go on to develop Borderline Personality Disorder? Why are some maltreated children not only haunted by the brutality and insensitivity they experienced but also grow to inflict similar abuse upon their own children, while others manage to interrupt the transgenerational transmission of abuse?

It is beyond the scope of this chapter to examine the burgeoning field of developmental psychopathology (see Cicchetti and Cohen 1995). A point of convergence is the notion that the crucial protective factor against biological or environmental misfortune is found in the context of the attachment system. Developmental and neurobiological research has drawn attention over the last decade to the biological preparedness of the human brain to be activated and organized by social interactions. Indeed, an abundance of evidence supports the view that only in a social-interactive environment can the brain mature and develop the capacities to regulate affects and create psychological experience. This biological preparedness is illustrated by the 'pre-wiring' of the normal neonate's brain to respond to the *absence* of people with a psychobiological response of alarm and hyperarousal. Likewise, the presence of human beings appears to elicit a biologically prepared 'down-regulation' of the alarm response (Kandel 1983). Human responsiveness is probably even more critical for vulnerable infants, for example the 'shy' infants described by Kagan (1994), as well as for infants constitutionally predisposed to intense hyperarousal and irritability.

Perry (1997) points out that the repeated failure of human response to the baby's signals of distress 'organizes' the developing brain in the direction of a proneness to full-blown 'fight or flight' reactions – which in the infant largely involves 'trance-like' states of dissociation.

Attachment theory (Bowlby 1973; Ainsworth *et al.* 1978) has offered a framework to investigate how the psychobiological regulatory functions of the human brain evolve in interactive systems in which the infant's signals of change in their subjective experience are understood and responded to by the caretakers. The infant's behaviour by the end of the first year of life appears purposeful and based on expectations generated by past experiences. Bowlby proposed that the aggregate of experiences with caretakers is organized by the infant into representational systems which he called *internal working models*. Internal working models allow infants to *anticipate* and develop coping strategies based on their expectations of other people's behaviour. These anticipatory and coping strategies are reflected in the attachment patterns first described by Ainsworth *et al.* (1978).

Infants classified as *secure* are those who readily explore the environment in the presence of the caretaker, are anxious in the presence of a stranger, are distressed during the caretaker's brief absences, but are quickly reassured and seek contact upon the return of the caretaker and promptly resume active exploration of the environment. The behaviour of secure infants is based on the experience of reported well co-ordinated and sensitive interactions with caretakers, which permit these infants to remain relatively organized even in stressful situations (Grossman *et al.* 1986; Sroufe 1996).

Prospective·longitudinal research has demonstrated the relative stability of attachment patterns across the life span. Securely attached children grow to become more resilient, self-reliant, socially oriented and more deeply connected with others (Sroufe 1983; Waters *et al.* 1979; Sroufe *et al.* 1990).

Over the last decade developmental research has sought to identify the specific protective factors embedded in – or provided by – a secure attachment. Along this line, developmentalists have drawn attention to a crucial, biologically ready capacity which has been referred to as mentalization, self-reflection, children's theories of mind or metacognitive monitoring. Mentalization is the universal capacity discernible even in very young children to discriminate human behaviour and interpret it in terms of putative mental states. This developmental acquisition permits children to respond not only to other people's behaviour but to their own grasp – or conception – of others' beliefs, feelings, attitudes, desires, hopes, pretence, intentions, plans, and so on. This capacity should not be confused with conscious insight – much less with an ability to explain other people's motives – but involves the instantaneous, moment-to-moment ability to 'read' an interpersonal situation in terms of the mental states underlying human behaviour. By attributing mental states to others, children make people's behaviour meaningful and predictable and thus can more effectively anticipate others' actions. As children can assess the meaning of other people's behaviour, they become capable of flexibly activating, from the multiple sets of internal working models they have organized on the basis of prior experience, the one(s) best suited to respond adaptively to a particular interpersonal transaction.

Exploring the meaning of others' actions, in turn, is critically linked with children's self-reflective ability to label and experience as meaningful their own psychic experiences, an ability that underlies the capacities for affect regulation, impulse control, self-monitoring and the experience of self-agency, that is, the sense of 'ownership' over one's own behaviour (Carlsson and Sroufe 1995; Gergely and Watson 1996).

By contrast, children with either chronic or intermittent failures of mentalization are unable to respond flexibly and adaptively to the symbolic, meaningful qualities of other people's behaviour. Instead, these children find themselves trapped in fixed, concrete patterns of interpretation and response – affect and motoric patterns of response that are not amenable to reflection or modulation. Arguably, the key feature of borderline children is an *intermittent* loss or retreat from mentalization in the context of specific cues within their attachment system.

An impressive body of research by Fonagy *et al.* (Fonagy, Steele and Steele 1991) is establishing the link between the development of mentalization and the presence of attachment figures – caretakers who have responded sensitively to the infant's signals – who treat the child as an intentional being. That is, the environmental trigger that activates the biologically prepared capacity to read social cues appears to be caretakers who respond to the infant's signals with behaviour that assumes that a mental state of need, desire, feeling, intention, etc. underlies the infant's behaviour. Thus, when caretakers 'make sense' of the child's behaviour and 'answer', for example, a child's cry with soothing, comforting behaviour *and* a verbal and non-verbal message – 'oh honey, you are so hungry' – they provide the cues that activate the inborn capacity to grasp that mental states underlie behaviour. In the behaviour of the caretaker the infant discovers his *own* as well as other people's subjectivity – a finding that echoes Winnicott's statement that the baby finds himself reflected in his mother's face (Winnicott 1965).

This discovery soon leads infants to realize that grasping and communicating meaning is the most effective strategy available for humans to relate and cope with adaptive demands. Research (Fonagy *et al.* 1996; Steele *et al.* 1996) is also beginning to demonstrate that the capacity to mentalize not only permits the individual to cope better with vulnerability and misfortune but also ensures the transgenerational transmission of this protective capacity: parents' mentalizing ability assessed before their children's birth strongly predicts the children's security of attachment and subsequent mentalization capacity.

Pathological development of mentalization and Borderline Personality Disorder

Maltreated children are at significantly higher risk of suffering an impairment in the development of mentalization (Schneider-Rosen and Cicchetti 1984; 1991; Beeghly and Cicchetti 1994; Cicchetti and Beeghly 1987). Maltreated infants are very likely to develop a *disorganized/disoriented* pattern of attachment, consisting of an erratic mixture of clinging and avoidance of caretakers, as well as seemingly undirected behaviour such as hand-clapping and head-banging and trance-like states of 'freezing' even in the presence of the caretakers (Main and Solomon 1990; Cicchetti and Beeghly 1987; Main and Hesse 1990).

Maltreatment, of course, does not occur in isolation, but as part of a family climate often characterized by chaos, neglect and emotional violence, an interpersonal context where the attunement to the child's inner states needed to 'trigger' the development of mentalization is often in short supply.

Particularly pernicious for the development of mentalization seem to be instances in which the children's signals of distress are traumatic reminders for the parents and evoke either the need to escape – and thus neglect – or a 'fighting' response to destroy the noxious stimuli, i.e. abuse. One mother, for example, reported how her baby's cry evoked in her uncontrollable panic, a need to get away and an overwhelming need to get the baby to 'shut up'. She would resolve her predicament by locking herself in the bathroom and then turning on the shower to muffle the inconsolable – and unattended – cries of her baby. Westen (1990) confirms the general validity of the case with the finding that infant's crying was given as the reason for child abuse by 80 per cent of mothers who abuse their children. Typically, an episode of abuse and/or neglect is followed by intense involvement, setting the stage for the disorganized/disoriented attachment pattern shown by as many as 80 per cent of abused infants and children.

Disorganized/disoriented attachment may represent the only coping strategy available to young children whose distress evokes parental 'fight or flight' – instead of the normal protective and comforting behaviour, coupled with parental responses that suggest that the parent is reacting to his/her 'read' of the child's mental state. Children 'retreat' from mentalization – the ongoing give and take of signalling one's mental states and 'reading' others' mental states that is the hallmark of secure attachment and a likely condition of optimal development – in response to their own states of distress when they identify that their distress evokes in the caretakers a terrifying mental state, that is, a desire to destroy them and/or run away from them. As Main and Hesse (1990) hypothesized, caretakers of disorganized/disoriented infants frequently respond to the infant's emotional distress with frightened and/or frightening behaviour. In effect, the infant's emotional expression triggers in the caretaker a temporary failure to perceive the infant as an intentional person.

The chaotic and contradictory features of approach and avoidance of the disorganized/disoriented pattern may represent not only the children's efforts to distance themselves from the awareness of their caretakers' mental states, but also the adaptation to the caretakers' usual behaviour following an abusive and/or neglectful episode: an anxious, guilt-ridden, overstimulating re-engagement and overinvolvement.

In the model proposed here, children on the path to developing a borderline personality are those who early on in their lives respond to parental misattunement and abuse with a 'fractionation' (Fischer *et al.* 1990) or splitting of mentalization across domains of interpersonal interaction.

These children come to experience their own arousal as a danger signal for abandonment – not concrete physical abandonment but what is probably even more pernicious from the standpoint of what the human brain requires for optimal functioning and growth: a human context that recognizes and responds to intentionality and mental states.

Thus, while they remain aware and are often hypersensitive and inordinately vigilant of others' mental states, in emotionally charged interactions future borderline children withdraw from a mentalizing stance. At that point, they are temporarily bereft of the adaptive capacity that a mentalizing function affords, i.e. they struggle (a) to maintain a stable and coherent sense of self; (b) to feel themselves as agents of their own behaviour; (c) to self-soothe and otherwise label, contain and regulate their affective experience; (d) to create a sense of direction and an ability to set self-limits and tolerate frustration; (e) to experience others as intentional beings and thus to feel *connected* to others through the mutual sharing of mental (meaningful) states.

Over time, children develop coping mechanisms to deal with the experiences of shattered security, subjective dyscontrol and emotional disconnection from others that accompany the loss of mentalization. These strategies become progressively more rigid and give shape to persistent maladaptive patterns of relating and organizing experiences that qualify for the designation of borderline personality.

Thus, borderline children gradually transform their sense of subjective dyscontrol and associated conviction that misery, passivity and helplessness will befall them into the active pursuit of self-victimization. Paradoxically, self-victimization induces a secret sense of power and control as these children no longer wait passively for abuse or victimization to happen to them, but skilfully evoke them.

Borderline children also become adept at actively creating states of numbness and dissociation when they fear becoming overwhelmed. Terr (1991), for example, describes a boy who coped with his step-father's brutal assaults by producing a self-hypnotic state in which he visualized himself sitting on his mother's lap while having a picnic at a beautiful park.

A subset of borderline children are particularly prone to dissociation and numbness which they experience as a terrifying sense of deadness. The role of a constitutional proclivity to dissociation is unclear. There is conflicting evidence that sexual abuse, particularly when severe, prolonged, accompanied by force or violence and perpetrated by a caretaker, is powerfully connected with the development of dissociative symptoms (Chu and Dill 1990; Zweig-Frank and Paris 1997). Feeling 'dead inside', these borderline children often experiment with self-mutilation and parasuicidal behaviour, which are meant to evoke feelings that will restore a sense of being alive. But self-mutilation also becomes an effective manoeuvre to secure attention and involvement from others while safely expressing anger. Veiled expressions of anger are necessary because of the 'fractionation' of the children's functioning: in the light of the caretaker's contradictory attitudes – and the loss of a mentalizing interaction under some circumstances (see above) – these children *split* their mental representation of the caretakers – and of themselves – into several coherent subsets.

Clinical studies (Putnam and Trickett 1997) suggest that the presence of dissociative symptoms is associated with more severe maladjustment and poorer response to treatment. But even those borderline children less inclined to dissociation – by biological predisposition and/or traumatic experience – strive mightily to numb themselves with food or drugs when threatened with the hyperarousal and panic they experience in intense interpersonal situations or when fearing abandonment and loss.

Some qualifications: biological vulnerabilities and trauma

The interaction of biological vulnerabilities, trauma and deficits in mentalization is unclear. Certain biological vulnerabilities such as attention deficit/hyperactivity or learning disorders are likely to limit children's evolving mentalizing capacities. This effect, like most aspects of development, creates a bi-directional process: biological vulnerabilities provoke interpersonal conflict and frustration as well as inherently limiting children's capacities. Thus, biological factors can limit the development of mentalization by generating environments which fail to promote it.

Of particular interest is the recent research on the psychobiological factors underlying PTSD. As Yehuda (1997) points out, PTSD occurs only in individuals who present a particular biological response to trauma which is neither typical nor normative.

Yehuda's research demonstrates that individuals who develop PTSD show *lower* than normal levels of cortisol, the hormone necessary to terminate the psychobiological response of hyperarousal and autonomic activation following a stressor. It appears that individuals predisposed to PTSD present an enhanced negative feedback inhibition of the hypothalamic–pituitary–adrenal axis. Chronic hypothalamic hyperstimulation of the pituitary leads to pituitary hyporesponsiveness, which in turn results in adrenal receptor hypersensitivity.

Thus, PTSD patients appear biologically predisposed to respond abnormally to stress, with both an inability effectively to terminate the brain's response to trauma (due to low basal levels of cortisol) *and* a subsequent hyperresponse to environmental challenges and traumatic reminders (due to hypersensitive adrenal receptors). Similar abnormalities have been identified in the sympathetic nervous system and other neuromodulatory systems (Shalev *et al.* 1993; McParlane *et al.* 1993; Murburgh 1994), and are consistent with the findings of hypervigilance, increased startle, irritability and physiological hyperarousal to traumatic reminders.

It is compelling to consider that some individuals present a biologic alteration *prior* to facing a traumatic event that shapes their response to trauma. Such biologic vulnerability may reflect a sensitization process due to an interaction of pre-existing risk factors – constitutional predisposition and environmental influences.

The model presented here proposes that some children are sensitized to respond catastrophically to stress and trauma by an unfavourable balance between constitutional vulnerability of neuromodulatory mechanisms and the protection afforded by the mentalization capacities produced in the context of secure attachment. This sensitization (a) increases the likelihood of subsequent stress and trauma by generating alienation and frustration in the children's interpersonal environment, and (b) decreases the opportunities to strengthen attachment and mentalization, thus further reducing the chance to acquire adaptive protective mechanisms against traumatization. As they face stress and trauma – particularly physical and/or sexual abuse – the sensitized children are thus prone to resort to the maladaptive characterological responses that mark the development of the borderline personality.

Treatment

Every intervention available to child and adolescent clinicians, from psychopharmacology to psychoanalytic psychotherapy, from behavioural approaches to family therapy, from special education to long-term residential treatment, has been advocated, backed mostly by anecdotal evidence and clinicians' theoretical convictions.

The central premise derived from the model presented in this chapter is that the crucial therapeutic goal for borderline children is the capacity to activate their ability to find meaning in their own and other people's behaviour even at times of stress, challenge or intense interpersonal demand.

To achieve this goal, the treatment needs to be intensive and multifaceted. Multiple and carefully integrated interventions are required to: (a) create an interpersonal context that provides effective limits to destructive behaviour – in the child and the family – while allowing for the recognition of mental states, and the enhancement of parental competence; and (b) develop an alliance and an attachment with the child that permits the examination of the child as an intentional being, including his or her intention to *retreat* – under some circumstances – from a mode of functioning that assumes intentionality in the self and in others.

Inpatient or residential treatment

Many borderline youngsters, particularly borderline adolescents, will, at one point or another, meet criteria for hospitalization; their behaviour – particularly suicidal or parasuicidal behaviour – is dangerous to self and/or others; their symptomatology continues to escalate in spite of outpatient interventions; or their aggression, impulsivity and manipulativeness become such a burden and elicit such harmful responses that hospitalization is sought to provide a 'cooling-off' period for the family.

A rich literature (e.g. Rinsley 1989; Bleiberg 1989) advocated long-term inpatient or residential treatment, claiming that months – if not years – in a controlled milieu were essential to overcome these children's pathological defences while allowing them to achieve genuine autonomy and self-regulation.

Extended residential treatment of the type proposed by Rinsley and Bleiberg has largely disappeared in the United States as managed care expanded its control over reimbursement and denied payment for anything but short-term crisis intervention.

While managed care limits have been driven by financial considerations, they served to stimulate more systematic scrutiny regarding the actual clinical effectiveness of the treatment approaches directed at borderline patients. Clinical studies with borderline adults (Linehan 1993; Chu 1998) are beginning to demonstrate that most borderline patients can be more effectively treated in settings that minimize regression and dependency, suggesting that only a minority of borderline children and adolescents may require extended residential treatment. Empirical studies are needed to delineate for which borderline youngsters extended residential treatment is indicated.

For most borderline youngsters inpatient or residential treatment aims to achieve the following goals: to stabilize an acute crisis; to promote an alliance with the caretakers and develop a long-term treatment plan; and to initiate a process that establishes the adults, both parents and treaters, as competent, effective and reliable protectors and limit-setters.

A context in which the caretakers can more effectively establish generational boundaries and block their children – and themselves – from automatic enactment of impulsive, manipulative and non-mentalizing behaviour appears to be a precondition for initiating a long-term therapeutic process focused on enhancing the child's mentalization.

Psychopharmacology is another crucial facilitator of mentalization by targeting specific symptoms which directly impair it, promote chaos and dysfunction in these children's environment, and further contribute to maladjustment. Symptomatic improvements have been noted with anxiolytics, antidepressants, stimulants, antipsychotics, mood stabilizers and anticonvulsants. Judiciously utilized, psychopharmacological agents can decrease impulsivity, anxiety and hyperarousal; improve attention and mood; and lessen cognitive distortions.

Individual treatment

There is wide consensus among clinicians working with borderline youngsters that the central aim of the beginning phase of therapy is to promote in the patient the notion that a collaborative activity with the therapist is possible, safe and potentially helpful.

Borderline youngsters can fall madly in love with their therapist. On the other hand, therapists may contend with an opening phase marked by ruthless tyranny, suspiciousness, demands for control of the sessions, or attempts to reduce the therapist's role to that of a captive audience of an elaborate show. Impulsive children may turn aggressive and destructive, and those who have experienced chronic trauma often present concrete, repetitive, joyless play.

Therapists must clarify limits from the beginning and provide structure when necessary. The process of enhancing mentalization is initiated by interventions focused on monitoring patients' affects and clarifying their subjective experience ('Let me see if I understand what you are saying'), with the goal of directing attention to a mentalizing perspective in which people recognize each other's mental states while helping patients feel that they can safely share, whether verbally or in play, at least some aspects of their experience. The therapist should avoid interpreting the patient's envy, sadness, vulnerability or rage as well as the associated defences of grandiosity, dissociation, denial and projection. It is important to discourage regressed, withdrawn and psychotic behaviour, and to clarify the difference between reality and fantasy. In line with this premise, therapists point to current moment-to-moment changes in the patient's mental states, refraining from attempting to link current mental states with conflictive, repressed or dissociated material.

When individual treatment is co-ordinated with family and day treatment, the therapist can facilitate the development of an alliance by helping the patient 'save face'. That is, therapists can help their patients maintain a sense of control when confronted with the caretakers' increasingly more effective limit-setting. Such interventions involve a delicate balance between fostering more adaptive solutions to reality's demands and keeping anxiety within manageable limits.

At the point when the patients give indications of experiencing a collaborative relationship, the therapist can gently encourage them to consider an expansion on the range of what is discussed in therapy. Borderline youngsters are introduced to the notion of continuity of the self and relationships.

As part of this process the therapist helps the patients understand both the conscious and unconscious relationship between their behaviour and internal states. The therapist makes explicit a mentalizing perspective when focusing patients' attention on the circumstances which led them, for example, to become aggressive when feeling misunderstood.

Yet only with the parents – and often a day programme's – assistance can the therapist attempt to explore and confront defences and the motives behind those defences. As borderline children face their vulnerability, they are filled with panic. Not surprisingly, a heightened reliance on old defences becomes apparent at this point in the therapy, i.e. efforts to control, intimidate, manipulate, or seduce the therapist, running away, drug abuse, self-mutilation, or attempts to pit parents and therapist against each other.

Therapists' acknowledgement of the difficulties involved in relinquishing familiar ways of coping can prevent stalemates and limit regression. If anything, therapists are on firmer ground when pointing out the advantages of *not* changing, that is, acknowledging the price patients pay when giving up their usual strategies for dealing with stress and conflict, however maladaptive these may be. Implicitly or explicitly, the decision the therapist outlines involves a choice between preserving the sense of control and safety provided by old defences and attempting to negotiate the laborious process of achieving real mastery and meaningful relationships.

This dilemma can often be better addressed in the 'transitional space' (Winnicott 1953) of play or humour. Playful, humorous, or fantasy scenarios provide an 'as-if' area where patients can both own and disown threatening internal states, feelings, thoughts and intentions while testing out the therapist's attunement, respect and responsiveness to the vulnerable aspects of the self. Kay Tooley's 'Playing it right' (1973) is an account of how the therapist can attempt to align borderline children's play and fantasy more closely with reality's constraints. This transitional space – shared play or a story jointly created by patient and therapist – becomes a stage on which to try out new identifications, to explore different ways of being in the world and relating to others, to practise imagined solutions to life dilemmas, and to test behaviour that promises greater mastery, more effective coping and increased pleasure and adaptation. In particular, play, humour and fantasy offer the magic of anonymity where the concrete can be seen as symbolic and where it becomes possible to 'play' at bringing together split-off representations of self and others. For abused children, the adult world is too real a threat to permit play. Yet the capacity to take a playful stance may be a critical step in the development of mentalization as it requires holding in mind simultaneously two realities, the pretend and the actual, in synchrony with a moment-to-moment reading of the other person's state of mind.

In the safe haven of the transitional space, the therapist can systematically explore the youngsters' defences and the motives for such defences. Gradually, patients are nudged to introduce small modifications in their play – and thinking – the better to encompass the complexities, limitations, conflicts and frustrations of reality.

Enhancing parental competence and sensitivity

Enduring changes in mentalizing capacities, and the readiness to relinquish rigidly held coping and relationship patterns, are unlikely unless such changes are syntonic with changes in children's interpersonal context.

Parental capacity to promote their children's mentalizing abilities involves an enhancement in their ability to consider and trust their children as intentional beings, endowed with a mind and life of their own. Such capacity, in turn, is predicated on the caretakers receiving help to feel more competent and in control, rather than buffeted by the emotional and behavioural turmoil they and their children generate. Thus, key aspects of the work with the parents are aimed at helping them become more effective and consistent limit-setters, more capable of introducing generational boundaries, and more invested in extricating their children from the special roles they often play within the family, detouring one parent's hostility against the other; holding the parents' marriage together; or maintaining parental self-esteem while relieving them from traumatic memories of pain, vulnerability and helplessness.

Analogous to children's intrapsychic adjustment, the family's patterns of coping and relating, however painful and maladaptive, have evolved to provide the best possible measure of safety and predictability. It is thus critical to begin treatment by establishing a therapeutic alliance with the parents based on a shared understanding of the children's difficulties and a clear agreement regarding the therapeutic steps needed to address those difficulties, as well as an understanding of the cost the family will incur in undertaking those steps.

From a family systems perspective, the diagnostic formulation provides treaters and parents with a common ground that gives the parents a historical, multigenerational context in which to look at the development of dysfunctional patterns of family interaction; avoids siding with one parent against the other or exacerbating parental guilt, shame or sense of incompetence; highlights children's role in maintaining and reinforcing dysfunction in the family every bit as much as the part played by dysfunctional family interactions in maintaining and reinforcing children's difficulties; defines the children's problems in terms of issues addressed by changing the way people interact with one another; and makes explicit that, whatever the nature of children's conflicts and anxieties, a major goal of treatment is to assist parents in being both in charge and more comfortable with parenting their children – rather than casting the therapist in the role of a new, more competent substitute parent.

Working with the parents gives the therapist access to a vantage point from which to assess the consequences to the family of the children's relinquishment of symptoms and the particular stresses that children's changes may trigger within the family. Working collaboratively with the parents serves to address a major source of resistance to treatment: children's anxiety that their growth and change will shatter the family and cause the parents to hurt one another, divorce, commit suicide, or abandon the child.

Children's involvement in treatment, in turn, characteristically mobilizes parental efforts, often unconscious, to undermine such engagement. From this point on, family therapy or individual therapy for one or both parents may be required. More typically, parental resistance can be addressed with a consistent respect for the parents' position as the ones who determine whether the treatment 'makes sense'.

Increasing parental capacity to express concerns directly and give and receive support and nurturance helps address the parents' feelings of exhaustion and depletion. Empathy for the children's plight, without increasing parental guilt, can be promoted, for example, by encouraging one or both parents to tell stories to their children about times when they felt distressed in circumstances comparable to those now faced by the children and how they coped with such distress. Story-telling can serve to connect parents with their own vulnerability in the process of helping their children and collaborating with the therapist rather than placing themselves in the role of patients.

Interventions with the parents change transactions within the family and, in so doing, not only improve children's developmental opportunities but also give children 'permission' to bring to the individual sessions a host of important issues, with greater freedom from the binds of loyalty or concern about the implied rules of family life.

Chapter 3

Mentalization and personality disorder in children

A current perspective from the Anna Freud Centre[1]

Peter Fonagy and Mary Target

There has been general agreement on the indications for child analysis. Anxious, inhibited, neurotic children are thought clinically to be particularly suitable. Glenn (1978), Sandler *et al.* (1980), Hoffman (1993), Paulina Kernberg (1995) and others have identified further criteria:

1 Superior intelligence, particularly verbal skills and psychological mindedness.
2 A supportive and stable environment, including parents who can form an alliance with the analyst, respect the boundaries of the treatment, and support their child's participation in it.
3 Internal conflict, judged to be the primary cause of the child's symptoms.
4 An absence of major ego deviations, that is, developmental 'deficits' that are not the result of unconscious conflict and thus cannot be 'resolved' by insight.
5 Motivation to engage in a lengthy and sometimes difficult therapy, stemming from anxiety, guilt or shame.
6 A capacity to form relationships, and trust that help can be found in relationships with others.

Few cases encountered in current clinical practice, certainly in the public domain, meet these stringent criteria. Their problems are mostly far more severe, emerge in the context of minimal inner resources and a background of chaotic and often persecutory hostile home environments. Can we expect child analysis to offer anything to these children?

An effort to answer this question was the chart review and detailed examination of over 750 case records of children and adolescents in psychoanalysis and psychodynamic treatment at the Anna Freud Centre (Target 1993; Target and Fonagy 1994a; 1994b; Fonagy and Target 1994; 1996b). Our study revealed that psychodynamic treatment was particularly effective for groups of children whose diagnosis included an emotional disorder. Over 80 per cent of children with a single diagnosis of an emotional disorder and relatively high levels of adaptation, that is, those closest to what the child analytic literature considers optimal candidates for child analysis, showed reliable improvement. Surprisingly, however, they appeared as likely to benefit from non-intensive therapy – one to two sessions per week – as from intensive – four to five sessions per week – treatment. Even more surprising was the finding that intensive treatment was remarkably effective for some children with relatively severe, long-standing and complex psychosocial problems, including Conduct Disorder, given the presence of at least one emotional disorder diagnosis – Anxiety Disorder, Dysthymia, etc. This heterogeneous group of children with complex psychopathology – which include children with borderline pathology – was less likely to gain clinically significant change from non-intensive psychotherapy. Even more disturbing was our observation that nearly 60 per cent showed negative outcomes following once- or twice-weekly treatment (Fonagy and Target 1996b).

Ongoing detailed analysis of our therapeutic records is revealing further suggestive findings. The most helpful interventions for the cases with more complex disorders seem to differ from those previously described as central to child psychoanalytic technique. In particular, interpretations of unconscious conflict aimed at promoting insight – long held as the centrepiece of analytic technique – appear of limited value to these youngsters. Less severely disturbed youngsters with emotional disorders, on the other hand, seem to benefit from an interpretative approach.

We are in the process of replicating these findings with young adults, 18–25-year-old young people with more than two Axis I and at least one Axis II diagnoses, assigned to five times or once weekly treatment. Although the results of the project, led by Mrs Anne Marie Sandler, are only in the process of being analysed, it is clear that once-weekly treatment appears frequently to contribute to a deterioration of these young people's condition, while five times weekly treatment has moderate to good therapeutic effects.

Based on these initial findings, the aim of this chapter will be threefold. First, we shall identify and describe the core disturbance which in our view characterizes children with 'mixed psychopathology'. Second, we shall offer a theoretical analysis of the nature of this core disturbance and provide some empirical support for our ideas. Third, we shall suggest a technical focus for analytic work with this unusual group of children.

Core disturbance in children with 'mixed psychopathology'

In our chart review the children with 'complex psychopathology' that appeared to benefit from intensive psychodynamic therapy constituted a rather heterogeneous lot, not easily captured by *DSM-IV*'s diagnostic categories. These children generally present a severe disturbance of social and emotional development, including marked impairment of peer relationships, affect regulation, frustration tolerance and self-image. With child-psychiatric input from Dr Efrain Bleiberg we have suggested that two clusters of such severe and complex problems could be discerned (Bleiberg *et al.* 1997). Cluster A children showed fragile reality contact and thought organization; idiosyncratic, magical thinking pervaded their lives, but acquired greater intensity in emotionally charged contexts. They tended to retreat into an isolated world of bizarre fantasies, suspiciousness and social anxiety. Their abilities to 'make sense' of human exchanges and empathize with others were strikingly limited. They were often equally impoverished in their capacity to communicate, hampered by odd speech and inappropriate affect. Descriptively, they generally resembled a range of *DSM-IV* (American Psychiatric Association 1994) diagnoses that include schizotypal and schizoid personality disorders, and milder forms of pervasive developmental disorder. They also resembled the children described by Towbin *et al.* (1993) and Cohen *et al.* (1994) as showing 'multiple complex developmental disorder'.

By contrast, a second cluster of children, which we have designated Cluster B, showed intense, even dramatic affect and hunger for social response. Clinginess, hyperactivity and temper-tantrums were common features of their early development. By school age, they commonly met diagnostic criteria for Attention-Deficit Hyperactivity Disorder, Conduct Disorder, Separation Anxiety Disorder or Mood Disorder. Many appeared anxious, moody, irritable, perhaps explosive. This affective lability mirrored the kaleidoscopic quality of these children's sense of self and others. One moment they felt elated, in harmony with an idealized partner. But at the next moment, they plunged into bitter rage, self-loathing or despair.

By the time they reached adolescence, drugs, food or promiscuous sex became common strategies to block feelings of subjective dyscontrol, fragmentation and loneliness. Self-mutilation and suicidal gestures were common among girls while aggression, coupled with hidden fears of rejection, was more typical of boys. We have some evidence to suggest that, if analysts are successful in maintaining Cluster B children in treatment, their outcome is comparable to that of children with neurotic disorders. Children in Cluster A generally have a poorer outcome, although they were less likely to terminate prematurely.

Undoubtedly, no single pathogenic factor can explain the heterogeneous subgroup of the children who may be considered as suffering from personality disorder with co-morbid severe emotional disorder. Constitutional vulnerabilities interact in various combinations with developmental factors, such as chronic illness or disability in the child, early parental loss, parental psychiatric disturbance, abuse and neglect, or restriction of autonomy. In spite of the heterogeneity, these youngsters seem to share a characteristic which we think is crucial and which we would like to focus on. Some pervasively (Cluster A) and others intermittently (Cluster B) seem to lack an essential developmental achievement: *the capacity to make use of an awareness of their own and other people's thoughts and feelings*. This capacity is referred to as 'mentalization' or 'reflective function', by both cognitive developmentalists (Morton and Frith 1995) and psycho-analysts (Fonagy 1991; Fonagy and Target 1995). It is maintained by neural structures which Simon Baron-Cohen and others have termed 'theory of mind mechanisms' (Baron-Cohen 1995) and localized with functional Positron Emission Tomography scans to the frontal lobe.

Mentalization or reflective function is the developmental acqui-sition that permits children to respond not only to another person's behaviour but to their *conception* of others' attitudes, intentions, or plans. Mentalization enables children to *'read' other people's minds*. By attributing mental states to others, children make people's behaviour *meaningful* and predictable. As children learn to understand other people's behaviour, they can flexibly activate, from the multiple sets of self–object representations they have organized on the basis of prior experience, the one(s) best suited to respond adaptively to particular relationships. Exploring the meaning of others' actions, in turn, is crucially linked with children's ability to label and find meaningful their own psychic experiences, an ability which underlies affect regulation, impulse control, self-monitoring, and the experience of self-agency.

To appreciate the nature of this developmental process we have to differentiate between two levels of mental functioning, not often distinguished in psychoanalysis. All mind is representation, but representations are themselves represented in the mind. In cognitive science, this is referred to as the distinction between cognition and metacognition. Some analytic authors (e.g. Freud 1911a; 1914; Segal 1957) who contrast the symbolic with concrete representations touch on a similar dimension. The deficit or dysfunction we are addressing here is at the level of metarepresentations. We believe that patients with certain severe personality disorders have no reliable access to an accurate picture of their own mental experience, the representation of their representational world. Thus, children with limited mentalization or reflective abilities are disadvantaged in social interactions. They are unable to 'take a step back' and respond flexibly and adaptively to the *symbolic, meaningful* qualities of other people's behaviour. Instead, these children find themselves caught in fixed patterns of attribution, rigid stereotypes of response, non-symbolic, instrumental uses of affect – mental patterns that are not amenable to either reflection or modulation.

Most modern psychoanalytic theories of self-development (e.g. Fairbairn 1952; Winnicott 1960a; Kohut 1977; Fonagy and Target 1997; Target and Fonagy 1996) assume that the psychological self (the part of the self-representation where the self is represented not as a physical entity but as an intentional being with goals based on thoughts, beliefs and desires) develops through one's perception of oneself (in another person's mind) as feeling and thinking (Davidson 1983). It is assumed that the parent who cannot think about the child's particular experience of himself[2] deprives him of a core of self structure which he needs to build a viable sense of himself. We suggest that developmental personality disturbances arise first of all from the child's failure to find his own mind, his experience of himself as a thinker of thoughts, believer of ideas, feeler of emotions, in the mind of the caregiver (see Fairbairn 1952).

We assume that, for the infant, internalization of this image performs the function of the 'containment of mental states' (Bion 1962a), which Winnicott has described as 'giving back to the baby the baby's own self' (Winnicott 1967b: 33). Through the internalization of these perceptions the infant begins to learn that his mind is not a direct replica of the real world but a version of it. The experience of containment involves the presence of another being who not only reflects the infant's internal state, but re-presents it as a manageable image, as something which is bearable and can be understood. The perception of self in the mind of the other becomes the representation of the child's experience, the representation of the representational world.

To give an example – like all emotion, anxiety for the infant is a confusing mixture of physiological changes, ideas and behaviours. When the mother reflects, or mirrors, the child's anxiety, this perception organizes the child's experience, and he now 'knows' what he is feeling. The mother's re-presentation of the infant's affect (her mirroring and other reflections to it) is internalized and becomes the higher-order representation of the child's experience. If the mirroring is too accurate, the perception itself can become a source of fear and it loses its symbolic potential. It is too fear-provoking to be internalized as the representation of the affect state, which will therefore remain diffuse and persist. We may presume that individuals for whom the symptoms of anxiety signify catastrophes (e.g. heart attack, imminent death, etc.) have metarepresentations of their primary emotional responses which are ineffective in containing their intensity through symbolization, perhaps because the original mirroring by the primary caregiver exaggerated the infant's emotions. If it is absent, not readily forthcoming, or is contaminated with the mother's own preoccupation, the process of self-development is even more profoundly compromised. In these instances the child internalizes an image which is out of synchrony with his experience; the metarepresentation of anxiety is then alien to the experience – a part of the experiential self that does not match the internal experience to which it is connected. We shall return to this pathogenic pattern below.

Admittedly, this is a speculative model but it is also empirically testable and might help answer the thorny question of why individuals with panic disorders consistently attribute immense significance to physiologically relatively mild levels of disequilibrium. In collaboration with Dr György Gergely, we are in the process of designing a series of studies of the infant's emotional understanding which will more directly test these ideas. In recent studies we have confirmed that mothers who soothe their distressed 8-month-old babies most effectively, following an injection, rapidly reflect the child's emotion; but this mirroring is 'contaminated' by displays of affect which are incompatible with the child's current feeling (humour, scepticism, irony and the like) which reflect coping, metabolization or containment. In displaying such 'complex affect' they ensure that the infant recognizes their emotion as analogous, but not equivalent, to his experience, and thus the process of symbol formation can begin.

We believe that the security of attachment between infant and caregiver is the critical mediator. A secure bond is one where the infant's signals are accurately interpreted by the caregiver, thus giving them meaning in terms of the caregiver's response. Normal affect regulation develops from the expectation of re-equilibration following arousal, through physical proximity to the object. The infant's signal of distress and the caregiver's coping/mirroring are combined into a single representation which comes to signify distress and becomes a critical part of the child's capacity to autoregulate emotion.

But what of the child whose caregiver totally fails to mirror the infant's internal state? Missing the normal experience of reflection of his own mental states, the child is most likely to take as the core of his psychological representation of himself the caregiver's distorted and often barren picture of the child. The child who fails to develop a representation of an intentional self is therefore likely to incorporate in his image of himself the representation of the other, sometimes mental, sometimes physical. The picture of the self will then be distorted, and the child's experience of himself is overly influenced by his early perceptions of what others think and feel, and strangely out of touch with what he himself or others are currently experiencing. We believe, along with Edith Jacobson (1964), that prior to the establishment of firm boundaries between representations of self and other, the infant's perception of the other comes to be internalized as part of that representational domain which will eventually become the reflective part of the self.

Many of these children show apparent failures of object permanence, leading to primitive separation anxiety or feelings of merger or fusion with the object. In reality, they continue to depend existentially on the physical presence of the other both for self-sustaining auxiliary metacognitive function (to continue to seek and find their intentionality in the mind of the other) and, more subtly, as a vehicle for the externalization of parts of the self-representation which are experienced as alien and incongruent with the self. This is why it is essential, as Winnicott (1967b) pointed out, that the mother acts in harmony with the infant's self, sometimes even to the detriment of or even the temporary abolition of her own self as an entity. If the other is consistently incongruent with the state of self, her presentation is still internalized as part of the self structure, but without the appropriate links and associations which would enable a coherent functioning of the infant's self-representation (Fonagy and Target 1997).

The ultimate consequences of this process can later be clearly discerned, we suggest, in borderline personality structure. In order for the self to be coherent, the alien and unassimilable parts require externalization; they need to be seen as part of the other where they can be hated, denigrated, even destroyed. The physical other who performs this function must remain present for this complex process to operate. This need for the other is related to but is qualitatively different from attachment behaviour as Bowlby (1969) described it. The borderline child or adult cannot feel that he is a self unless he has the other present (often the analyst) to frighten and intimidate, to seduce and excite, to humiliate and reduce to helplessness. There is, however, no attachment to the other, in terms of a serious expectation that the other may act in ways that regulate arousal. There is abandonment anxiety but it is not linked to the specific figure of the therapist (who is intrinsically neither loved nor hated). The other's departure signals the return of these 'exterojects' and the destruction of the coherence the child achieves by such projection. The other's departure signals the potential loss of the self.

This process, we believe, is also at the root of that type of projective identification where the patient feels an overriding need to control the other, as its self is only actualized when the other's behaviour can be forced to be consistent with this projective process. For example, a 9-year-old boy's mother permitted him to treat her as an extension of himself both physically and psychologically. In the analysis, he had to resort to far cruder devices, revealing the same underlying need. He frequently tied his analyst up, as well as constantly ordering her to do things for him. In our view, with cases as severely impaired as this child was, understanding such behaviour as an extension of the eroticized transference is unlikely to be helpful. In this case, what turned out to be important was the child's need to make the therapist's thoughts and feelings (of rage, hatred, disgust, helplessness) predictably present, and to eliminate other ideas or feelings which the therapist presented to him (worry, anxiety, a sense of nameless dread), which were unrepresentative and therefore unpredictable and terrifying.

At the root of disturbance like that of this boy is, we suggest, a failure to achieve full mentalization of affect, which we see as the integration of two more primitive forms of representing psychic reality (Fonagy and Target 1996b; Target and Fonagy 1996).

The dual nature of early psychic reality and trauma

In early childhood, reflective function is characterized by two modes of relating internal experiences to the external situation: in a serious frame of mind, the child expects the internal world in himself and others to correspond to external reality, and subjective experience will often be distorted to match information coming from outside ('psychic equivalence mode') (e.g. Perner *et al.* 1987; Gopnik and Astington 1988). While involved in play, the child knows that internal experience may not reflect external reality (e.g. Bartsch and Wellman 1989; Dias and Harris 1990), but then the internal state is thought to have no relationship to the outside world, and to have no implications for it ('pretend mode').

In normal development the child integrates these two modes to arrive at the stage of mentalization, or reflective mode, in which mental states can be experienced as representations. Inner and outer reality can then be seen as linked, yet they are accepted as differing in important ways, and no longer have to be either equated or dissociated from each other (Gopnik 1993; Baron-Cohen 1995).

We have hypothesized that mentalization normally comes about through the child's experience of his mental states being reflected on, prototypically through experience of secure play with a parent or older child, which facilitates integration of the pretend and psychic equivalence modes, through an interpersonal process which is perhaps an elaboration of the complex mirroring of the infant by the caregiver. In playfulness, the caregiver gives the child's ideas and feelings (when he is 'only pretending') a link with reality, by indicating the existence of an alternative perspective, which exists outside the child's mind. The parent or older child also shows that reality may be distorted by acting upon it in playful ways, and through this playfulness a pretend but real mental experience may be introduced.

In traumatized children, intense emotion and associated conflict can be thought of as having led to a partial failure of this integration, so that aspects of the pretend mode of functioning become part of a psychic equivalence manner of experiencing reality. This may be because, where maltreatment or trauma has occurred within the family, the atmosphere tends to be incompatible with the caregiver 'playing with' the most pressing aspects of the child's thoughts; these are often disturbing and unacceptable to the adult, just as they are to the child. The rigid and controlling behaviour of the pre-school child with a history of disorganized attachment is thus seen as arising out of a partial failure on the part of the child to move beyond the mode of psychic equivalence in relation to specific ideas or feelings, so that he experiences them with the intensity that might be expected had they been current, external events.

The almost impossible challenge patients present is, we believe, rooted in this aspect of the transference. For the relationship to serve a function and to be tolerable, the analyst must do something fresh and creative, 'an act of freedom' (Symington 1983), which has as one component the real impact of the real patient on the analyst, yet through its novelty reassures the patient that his attempt at control and tyranny has not completely succeeded. Through identification with the externalized part of the patient's self, the analyst has validated the patient's psychic reality, yet, by bringing a new perspective, has forced him to see another dimension to his own action and thus overcome the one-to-one correspondence between thought and reality in his mind. Without such creative spark the analysis is doomed to become an impasse, a rigid stereotypic repetition of pathological exchanges.

The challenge is the preservation of the 'as-if' nature of the therapeutic exercise, and sometimes playfulness is the only ally.

A man with a violent disposition was greatly distressed by a rather clumsy interpretation made to him. Aiming to be empathetic, the analyst referred to the pain he felt about a cancelled session. The patient promptly got up, shoved his fist under the analyst's nose, and said, 'I'll show you what pain is, you little shit!' Without thinking, the analyst said, 'You know, as I get older I can't see things so clearly when they are too close to my eyes', and with that gently moved the clenched fist away from his face. To the analyst's relief and surprise, the patient immediately calmed down and smiled. On reflection, the analyst realized what was critical to this exchange: forcing this patient to experience the world through the analyst's somewhat long-sighted perspective, and thus to see him as a real person, allowing the patient to enter his mental world.

Self, action and the body

Over ten years ago, Daniel Stern (1985) summarized findings and offered theories tracing self development back to the actions of the 4-month-old. A sense of authorship of one's own actions, whether derived from the experience of forming plans, proprioceptive feedback or the consequences of physical action, contributes to the continuity of the sense of self. Where actions are significantly curtailed, self agency and continuity are threatened. Bolton and Hill (1996), in their outstanding book *Mind, Meaning and Mental Disorder*, make a strong case for the 'close connection between thoughts and action, and of the experience of effective agency as crucial to the sense of self' (1996: 368). This crucial link of intentionality between thought and action cannot be totally sustained by the actions of the child, as these usually continue to be limited because of his immature physical and cognitive capacities, in certain respects until adolescence. Playful interpersonal interaction which permits the registration of perceptions, thoughts and emotions as causes and consequences of action, and the contemplation of these mental states without fear, provide the basis of self agency.

Coercive, rigid, frightening and, at an extreme, abusive parenting can undermine not just the understanding of mental states but also the establishment of a firm connection between the self and action, as this connection crucially depends on the perceived bi-directional link between mental state and action.

Disorders of conduct may be understood as the consequence of the child having failed to link his sense of self with his actions. In the case of abuse, the meaning of intentional states in terms of their truth value are also commonly compromised by the parent's denial of the child's internal reality. Abuse, particularly within the family, prevents the child testing representations of mental states for their applicability, truth and possible modification. They thus become rigid and unhelpful, and are partially and sometimes almost fully abandoned.

The experience of helplessness and defensive decoupling of painful bodily experiences associated with maltreatment may cause the individual to blame his body for the abuse. The body is less likely to be experienced as a potent agent of action, and actions on it are less integrated with the self. It is nonetheless perceived as the cause of difficulties, and thus action directed against it relieves both frustration and anger, the overriding goal being survival.

Another possible outcome is that the representation of the body may be used as if it were part of the psychic apparatus. In these cases the child's own body is used in representing and expressing feelings, ideas and wishes. It is therefore frequently attacked in desperate efforts to grapple with feelings and ideas. Boys commonly attack the body of the other to destroy the mental states they projected into them whilst girls attack their own bodies for analogous reasons. Young women with apparently uncontrollable insulin-dependent diabetes often fall into this group (Moran 1984; Fonagy and Moran 1993). In other young children, the search for the psychological self in the other may lead to the *physical* image of the object being internalized as part of the child's identity. The little boy then wishes to be a woman in order to be consistent with this introject, and gender identity disorder may be the consequence (Coates *et al.* 1991).

The decoupling of self-representation and action because of the disruption of the child's intentional stance is as relevant for violence against the other as for violence against the self. In conduct-disordered children, the broken link between action and psychological self is painfully clear, as those who have treated kicking and biting children would probably testify. A critical obstacle to interpersonal aggression, the innate responsiveness to another person's suffering through identifying with their state of mind, is lost. This is not, as is often claimed, to be attributed to the absence of empathy, although to be sure there is little evidence of this. Rather, violence reflects the absence of a critical precursor of empathy, a meaningful link between the self and the acts perpetrated by the body, the capacity to link action and mental state, which normally begets the psychological self.

Another consequence of the weak link between thinking or feeling and action is that violence or aggression may be resorted to as the only acts which succeed in linking intentional state to external events. Both violent and self-harming individuals feel real when attacking someone physically. We believe (Fonagy, Moran and Target 1993; Fonagy and Target 1995) that violent acts combine two powerful motivations for such people: the aggression and damage can lend a sense of coherence to the self (self-actualization), and at the same time it expresses the need to attack externalized, alien aspects of the self, either felt to be in one's own body or represented by somebody else.

Empirical support

There is a certain amount of empirical data, from experimental studies of the development of social cognition in normal and abnormal children, and from studies of parent–child attachment, which is consistent with this model.

As we mentioned, developmentalists for the most part refer to mentalizing as maintained by a theory of mind mechanism. Dennett (1978) convincingly argued that the understanding of mental states, such as belief, could only be unequivocally demonstrated by the individual showing an understanding that someone else could have a false belief. The capacity to mentalize is thus operationalized as the child being able to pass a false belief task, to show understanding that someone else would act or desire something based on a mental state the child knows to be mistaken. There is substantial accumulating evidence that theory of mind mechanisms (ToMM) are dysfunctional in children with autism (Baron-Cohen 1995).

We believe that lesser degrees of ToMM deficit, with a large psychosocial component, are prevalent in the group of children with developmental disturbances we have considered above. This suggestion fits the expectations of developmental psychologists working on the development of ToMM in normal children, who have explored the likely consequences of a child not 'discovering the mind' in the normal way – impairment of family and peer relationships, the capacity to learn, and emotional control (see, for example, Astington 1994: 146–7). A number of distinct lines of evidence converge to underline the plausibility of the model we are proposing.

In a programme of work over the last ten years several laboratories, including the London Parent–Child Project led by Miriam and Howard Steele, have been able to demonstrate the importance of the caregiver's capacity to think about their own past relationships in terms of their own and others' mental states to ensure the child's security of attachment (Fonagy, Steele, Moran *et al.* 1991). The presence of social deprivation in the mother's background greatly increases the importance of reflective capacity (Fonagy *et al.* 1994). The capacity to mentalize may permit the individual to cope with social trauma and disadvantage. The caretaker's efforts to make sense of the infant's behaviour convey to him that mental states underlie behaviour and that finding this meaning is the most effective strategy to relate and cope with the social environment. The child's sense of himself as an intentional being evolves to the extent that he can clearly perceive those intentions in the mind of the caregiver.

Studies of parent–child attachment have demonstrated that mentalization is a biologically prepared capacity *triggered* by an attachment figure who treats the child as an intentional being. A secure attachment relationship creates the emotional environment within which the child's opportunity to discover his intentional state, mentalizing capacity or theory of mind is maximized, and predicts ToMM (Fonagy *et al.* 1996).

In a number of clinical papers (Fonagy 1991; Fonagy and Target 1995), we have reported that individuals with features of borderline personality disorder appear to have specific difficulties in understanding mental states (both in themselves and in others) and that this dysfunction may be seen as an adaptation to intolerable experiences of maltreatment and abuse in childhood. Rather than contemplate the intolerable idea of what may be going on in the mind of their abuser, these children opt to inhibit their capacity to think about minds altogether, decouple the link between self-representation and action and turn away from the world of thoughts, feelings, beliefs and desires, at least in the context of intense attachment relationships. Studies of maltreated children show that they have both disrupted attachment (Cicchetti and

Barnett 1991) and a specific difficulty in acquiring mental-state words (Beeghly and Cicchetti 1994). Our studies of adult non-psychotic psychiatric inpatients show that those who have documented histories of severe maltreatment, with current significant impairments in understanding mental states, almost invariably meet DSM diagnostic criteria for Borderline Personality Disorder (Fonagy *et al.* 1996).

We are currently involved in prospective work at the Menninger Clinic to demonstrate that the difficulties of children with developmental disorders may be understood in terms of insecure attachment in infancy and the sequelae of this, which seem to include impairment in the full development of mentalizing. This, in turn, leaves them vulnerable to subsequent psychosocial stress (or may contribute to the generation of such stress), to which they respond by the sometimes dramatic inhibition of mentalizing function. It is our view that a metacognitive deficit brought about by psychosocial experiences, which undermines the healthy development of the ToMM, may account for self-regulation deficits (such as problems of affect regulation, frustration tolerance, impulsiveness and self-esteem problems), as well as social deficits (such as poor peer relationships, poor communication skills and aggressive or violent behaviour) (Bleiberg *et al.* 1997).

It is our premise that a *crucial* therapeutic aspect of psychoanalysis – for both children and adults – lies in its capacity to activate people's ability to find meaning in their own and other people's behaviour. Child psychoanalysis has always aimed at strengthening children's capacity to recognize mental states. We believe that a therapeutic programme that engages in a *systematic* effort to enhance mentalization holds the promise of increasing the effectiveness of psychoanalysis for the children with more severe and complicated difficulties, by more specifically tailoring therapeutic intervention to their particular configuration of clinical and developmental problems.

Clinical implications

So what does a child-analytic approach focused on enhancing mentalization look like? Work at the Anna Freud Centre over at least three decades has evolved a set of techniques for helping children with primarily developmental disturbances, or more borderline pathology, and our formulations began with studying this work in the records of completed cases. For now we shall consider only three aspects, which are covered at greater length in a recent paper (Bleiberg *et al.* 1997).

Enhancing reflective processes

How does one go about enhancing mentalizing capabilities? First, such patients need to learn to observe their own emotions – to understand and label their emotional states, including their physiological and affective cues. They need help to understand both the conscious and the unconscious relationships between their behaviour and internal states, for instance of frustration or anxiety.

As part of that process, the analyst focuses children's attention on the circumstances which lead them, for example, to be aggressive in particular situations in which they feel misunderstood or made anxious by those around. The analyst introduces a mentalizing perspective which focuses on children's minds, *as well as* the mental states of people who are important to them.

The focus is kept, at least initially, on simple mental states. These children are unable to accept complex mental states of conflict or ambivalence, but may understand simple states of belief and desire. They will typically fail to grasp how mental states may change over time. Thus, working with current, moment-to-moment changes in children's mental states within the therapy is crucial. Likewise, analysts generally refrain, early in the process, from linking children's feelings with dynamically unconscious thoughts. An individual who fails to recognize his subjective experience can hardly relate to an even more inaccessible realm. Of course, by definition, the analyst is always addressing a non-conscious realm, feelings and ideas, which the patient has limited capacity to become aware of.

Clinical experience has shown that some patients find it helpful to focus interventions around their perceptions of the analyst's mental states, as a precursor to self-reflection (Steiner 1994). They can get to know the way they are seen by others, which can then become the core of their own self-perceptions. Analysts, of course, do not necessarily reveal to the children what they actually experience; rather, they speculate about how a child might be experiencing his state of mind at that moment. Some analysts have used guessing games along these lines: 'What do you think I am thinking about you today?' (Moran, 1984).

Play helps children to strengthen impulse control and enhance self-regulation

Children with mentalizing problems tend to require considerable help in curbing impulsivity. Rosenfeld and Sprince (1965) described a 6-year-old child, Pedro, who frequently urinated over the analyst and her possessions. Other features of the material led the analyst to understand this as a crude attempt to coerce her into mutual activity, or simply to maintain a sense of connection. Neither interpretations nor physical restraint reduced the behaviour. The analyst then devised a way of meeting what she had felt to be his need by saying that she would continue with the interrupted joint activity while he went to the lavatory, and she would give him a running commentary on what she was doing while he was there. He then stopped urinating in the treatment room and was able to still feel in contact through her voice. Pedro's analyst identified the gap in mentalization that triggered impulsivity and compensated for it.

Cluster B children often seem *more* impaired in their impulse control and self regulation as their attachment to the analyst becomes more intense. The temporary impairment of mentalization appears linked to the activation of traumatic responses triggered by closeness and/or separation from attachment figures (Van der Kolk 1989; 1994; Van der Kolk and Fisler 1994; Terr 1994). For example, Joe, a 13-year-old boy, had been subjected to brutal physical and sexual abuse by an alcoholic father while his mother pursued her theatrical career. Almost in spite of himself, he began to feel more comfortable with the analyst, even to look forward to the sessions. Yet desires for closeness were almost unbearable for him; thus, he began to carefully look for 'mistakes' (e.g. the analyst interrupting him or 'invading' his space while walking). These would trigger hateful barrages. He let the analyst know of his plans to run away and find out the analyst's address ('I have good sources, you know') so that he could set the analyst's house on fire after raping his wife and murdering his children with slow, intravenous injections of cocaine. He would spare the analyst's life, but only to ensure that he would suffer the devastation of the loss of everything he held dear.

Sensing his desire to maintain a relationship, while overtly disowning it, the analyst commented on the meanness and cruelty of his imagery. Where did that come from? Joe looked at him with a mix of contempt and amusement and proceeded to describe, in a wildly exaggerated fashion, the toughness of his neighbour-hood and its brutal gang wars. He was sure that the analyst's wimpy, nerdy self had been shielded from such roughness. The analyst entered the role and created play. He replied with an even more fantastic account of his own heroic battles as a gang kingpin – a secret identity hidden behind his deceptively mild appearance. The banter continued over several sessions – but gradually the analyst was able to return Joe's attention to the rage he had experienced and the abuse he inflicted on the analyst.

This vignette illustrates how such youngsters often require a transitional area of relatedness akin to Winnicott's (1953) transitional experience. In this transitional, as-if area (often jointly created by patient and analyst) standing between fantasy and reality, patients can both own and disown their rejection feelings and experiences and test out the analyst's attunement, respect and responsiveness to the vulnerable aspects of the self. The essence of the interaction appears to be the provision of a safe context in which to play with ideas and come to experience them *as* ideas.

The patient's threat, even if it is verbal rather than physical, is experienced by him as action; its modulation by the analyst into an idea allows it to be played with, mentalized, thus creating the potential for understanding. For the abused child, the adult's mental world is too real a threat to permit play, and is thus shunned and avoided. The analyst's attitude and verbalization permit the opening of a window on the mental world of self and other, but the child has to find the courage to use this, to look through it and find his own feelings and ideas – something which has never before felt safe. In other words, the therapeutic intent is to facilitate the establishment of a beachhead, an area of self–other relatedness. Prematurely confronting the patient's defences before this beachhead is established only exacerbates the need for distance, control, or devaluation of the analyst and the therapy.

The capacity to take a playful stance may be a critical step in the development of mentalization as it requires holding simultaneously in mind two realities: the pretend and the actual, in synchrony with a moment-by-moment reading of the other person's state of mind. Analysts often need to create a context in which an attitude of pretence is possible. For example, they may exaggerate their intonations to mark for children the pretend nature of interactions, or may choose objects which are clearly incapable of adopting any intentional stance (crude toys, for example).

Gradually, children are nudged to introduce small modifications in their play the better to encompass the complexities, limitations, conflicts and frustrations of reality. The transitional space of play and fantasy offers borderline children the magic of anonymity in which to attempt to bring together split-off representations of the self and others.

Working in the transference

Finally, the emphasis is on working in the transference – not 'transference' in the classic sense of expecting children to 'transfer' their thoughts and feelings about their parents on to the analyst. What is externalized in these transferences is not an internal representation of a self–other relationship, but rather an unwanted alien part of the self. No relationship is experienced in this context except insofar as the child needs to manipulate the other so that she can fulfil the function of being a vehicle (a receptacle) for the repudiated aspects of the self-representation. Thus the relationship with the analyst remains central. The clarification of children's feelings about themselves and about the analyst is the most effective route towards acquiring mentalizing capacity.

The analyst uses her experiences with the child as a vehicle for helping the child to find, through involvement in a therapeutic relationship, a way of thinking, understanding and coping with feelings; of recognizing the connections and differences between oneself and somebody else, and of being with another person.

Accepting and recognizing the mental chaos of the child, and abandoning the traditional stance of recovering forgotten memories, is the first step in the process. The past makes no sense as a cause of the present, as it is the present that cannot be thought or felt about. The analyst has to teach the child about minds, principally by opening his mind to the patient's explorations of the analyst's internal world. '*Deep* interpretations' of unconscious wishes will be experienced as persecutory taunts, intrusions, distractions or seductions. The appropriate focus of work is the exploration of triggers for feelings, small changes in mental states, highlighting differences in perceptions of the same event, bringing awareness to what would be almost conscious for most people. Work takes place strictly in the analyst–patient relationship, and focuses on the mental states of patient and analyst. Interpretations are not global summaries but rather attempts at placing affect into a causal chain of concurrent mental experiences. The patient's actions on the analyst are not intended as communications (and interpreting them as such is therefore not appropriate). They are desperate attempts at coping with the intolerable closeness which analysis brings.

The analyst adopts a non-pragmatic, elaborative, mentalistic stance, which places a demand on the child to focus on the thoughts and feelings of a benevolent other. This stance, in and of itself, enhances, frees or disinhibits the patient's inborn propensity for reflection and self-reflection. Perhaps more important, he is able to find himself in the mind of the analyst as a thinking and feeling being, the representation that never fully developed in early childhood and was probably further undermined by subsequent painful interpersonal experience. In this way, the patient's core self-structure is strengthened and sufficient control is acquired over mental representations of internal states so that psychotherapeutic work proper can begin. Even if work were to stop here, much would have been achieved in terms of making behaviour understandable, meaningful and predictable. The internalization of the analyst's concern with mental states enhances the patient's capacity for similar concern towards his own experience.

Conclusion

Psychoanalysis is under savage attack in most countries where it is practised. Yet intensive psychosocial treatments for severe psychological disorders are increasingly seen as essential by clinicians with behavioural, cognitive and systemic orientations. We recommend a shift in analytic technique from a repression- and insight-oriented approach to a focused, mentalization-oriented therapy, which we believe is already widely used by those treating severe psychological disturbance. Psychoanalytic training, supervision and personal treatment remain crucial in enabling clinicians to use their emotional reactions to understand their patient's subjective world better, rather than be entrapped in the quicksand of rigid, unthinking patterns of relatedness without the possibility of reflection. The techniques suggested here and the theoretical ideas on which they are based may also be put to good effect in prevention, informing parenting training, home visitation programmes, nursery education and crime prevention initiatives.

The change of aims and priorities we are suggesting is not radically new or exclusive of other approaches, which of course include more classical technique with the 'good, neurotic case'. At its strongest, our claim is that severe disorders of character require modifications of technique in the direction of prioritizing a mentalizing approach. At its weakest, we are introducing new jargon into an area already bursting with terminological confusion. However, even here, there may be value added by harmonizing our language with that of developmental cognitive science.

We do believe that we are doing analysis with these patients, in that we are trying to understand the roots of psychological problems in early emotional development, encompassing the whole range of conscious and unconscious motivations, within the intense relationship with the analyst. Thus, we believe that we may contribute to the advancement of Freud's vision of development, psychopathology and therapeutic action.

Notes

1   A shortened version of this chapter was presented by the authors as the 1997 Marianne Kris Memorial Lecture at the Annual Meeting of the Association for Child Psychoanalysis Inc., March 1997, Cancún, Mexico. We would like to acknowledge the vital contributions of Dr Efrain Bleiberg and Drs Miriam and Howard Steele to the thinking and empirical work which are drawn on in this chapter.

  George Moran initiated a programme of work at the Anna Freud Centre, which, starting with the work on juvenile-onset diabetes (Fonagy, Steele, Moran *et al.* 1991), has led us to ask fundamental questions about the nature of the child psychoanalysis, with important implications for technique. We acknowledge our debt by dedicating this chapter to George Moran, whom we see as a worthy successor to Marianne Kris, both of them working within the tradition of Anna Freud.

2   For clarity, we have sometimes referred to the child as he, and to the caregiver or therapist as she. This makes it easier to follow, and corresponds to the actual gender in the large majority of instances.

Chapter 4

A developmental view of 'defence'

The borderline psychotic child

Anne Alvarez

The case of the borderline psychotic child, where there may be some ego development, although of only a minimal or fragile sort, raises similar problems to those in the treatment of the psychotic child. The diagnosis is unfortunately not widely used among child psychiatrists who are not psychoanalytically trained. It does not exist at all in the ninth or tenth editions of the *International Classification of Diseases* (*ICD*), and while it appeared in the third *Diagnostic and Statistical Manual* (*DSM-III*) of the American Psychiatric Association as a subcategory of personality disorder, this practice was dropped in *DSM-IV*.

I am using the term 'borderline psychotic' in a much wider sense to include the other subcategories of personality disorder such as compulsive, antisocial paranoid, schizoid and avoidant, and so on. The psychiatric classifiers are, I suppose, uncomfortable with too wide a use of the word 'psychotic' to describe children who are not flagrantly so, partly because the word still has pejorative associations in the lay (and organically minded psychiatric) mind. To the psychoanalytic psychotherapist, the notion of a psychotic part of the personality, or the evidence of (hopefully brief) instances of psychotic thinking, in everyone's life is perfectly comfortable, and so no more pejorative than the label 'personality disorder'. Furthermore, when the quality and level of anxiety is understood (along with the content and form of some of the phantasies), the word 'psychotic' attached to 'borderline' seems perfectly appropriate. It also has important implications for theory and technique in relation to such children.

Most writers in the field tend to describe adult borderline patients as existing on a continuum between psychosis and neurosis. This vertical dimension, which describes both the degree of pathology and the level of ego functioning, is useful as a rough guide in unknown territory, but it should not be allowed to narrow one's focus, for most of the writers are in fact referring to an extremely broad range of illness. The categories – on the horizontal axis, as it were – tend to include everything from the psychopathic character disorders through the immature personality, the narcissistic disorders, severe neurotic conditions with psychotic features, excessively severe depression, to what used to be called latent schizophrenia but would now more likely be termed borderline schizophrenia (LeBoit and Capponi 1979). The child psychotherapist might want to add many severely deprived, abused and traumatized children who have sometimes much in common with psychotic children, but in other respects are very different. They are different from borderline adults because psychotic illness in children, however temporary or however much only a threat from beyond the border, interferes with normal psychological development and therefore often produces developmental arrest and developmental deficit. When Kernberg (1975) describes the preponderance of primitive defences in the borderline patient, defences like splitting, idealization and devaluation, and projective identification, he is referring mainly to adults. But in children who are showing borderline disturbance we need to consider their pathology, and their use of primitive defences, as reflecting what is manageable by them in view of their deficit and vulnerability. In Kleinian terminology, of course, these primitive defences form part of the paranoid-schizoid position, and it is my purpose in this chapter to show that alongside the concept of defence we need a general concept of *overcoming* to reflect what is adequate or good enough about the steps the child takes to establish contact with the world.

Defences and developmental achievements or overcomings

Ornstein (1983) suggests it was probably a mistake over the years to think of deficit as a void that has to be filled, as Kohut (1977) implied. Kohut believed it was important to develop what he called the normal narcissistic pole of the personality and he has been much criticized for gratifying the idealizing narcissistic transferences. It has been claimed that he was doing supportive psychotherapy rather than analysis – what some writers would call manipulating the transference rather than analysing it. That seems to me to be another too simplistic dichotomy, which could be clarified by considering some of the problems that may arise from the psychoanalytic concept of defence. In Kleinian thinking, for example, a paranoid-schizoid patient may be defending himself against the truths of the depressive position – that is, against his love or his guilt – but he may also be suffering from impaired development, so that he cannot yet proceed to the depressive position.

This brings up a vital practical question: what are the conditions under which development forward is possible at any stage? These considerations must shape whether the therapist interprets a patient's suspiciousness or detachment as a defence against a closer and better relationship – which it may be – or whether it is understood as a protection against what he perceives to be a genuinely attacking or intrusive or useless object. For the chronic borderline case, who fluctuates back and forth between madness and sanity and where the amalgam of the psychotic part and the non-psychotic part may be very complex (see Grotstein 1979 and Steiner 1991), the technical situation can be very tricky indeed. It is important to know when obsessional mechanisms are being used defensively against an experience of a more living, free, less controllable object or feeling, and when they signal perhaps the very first attempt, or at the very least a renewed attempt, to achieve some slight order in the universe. It is important also to distinguish between the moments when a manic experience of an ideal object or an ideal situation is used as a defence against a more sober reality and when it signals the first glimmer of emergence from lifelong clinical depression. While Bion (1962a) has taught therapists to distinguish between mechanisms designed to modify frustration and those designed to evade it, Joseph's term 'psychic equilibrium' provides us with a concept much subtler than that of defence. In 'On understanding and not understanding' she writes, 'The patient who believes he comes to be understood actually comes to use the analytical situation to maintain his current balance in a myriad of complex and unique ways' (Joseph 1983: 142).

I have written elsewhere (Alvarez 1992: Ch. 10) about the fundamental theoretical and metatheoretical advance in the Kleinian differentiation between processes designed to defend against and processes designed to overcome depressive anxieties. I have come to think that a comparable distinction needs to be made when discussing the persecutory anxieties of the paranoid-schizoid position. I would like to consider in the present chapter those features of the paranoid-schizoid position that are viewed as 'classical' defences, namely, splitting, projection, projective identification, and idealization, and to discuss them from the perspective of their developmental origins and meanings.

The paranoid-schizoid position as a developmental phase

Klein first outlined her notions of the paranoid and depressive positions in two papers, 'Psychogenesis of manic-depressive states' (1935) and 'Mourning and its relation to manic-depressive states' (1940). It is probably well known that Klein did at first make some attempt to think in terms of phases and dates for these two very different states of mind – that is, she was thinking in terms of a developmental theory, following the tradition begun by Freud (1905) with his libido theory and continued by Abraham (1927). Gradually, however, the phase concept left Klein's writings altogether and she stuck much more closely to the notion of position. The idea of a position is, of course, a spatial metaphor and, in Klein's theory, it implied not just a different bodily location for the libido, but was, by definition, a relational – that is, an object-relational – term. In deference to Fairbairn, Klein added the schizoid concept to the paranoid position, and the characteristics at the schizoid end of the position are thought to be excessive splitting and fragmentation, excessive projection – later, in 1946, she added projective identification – a consequent weak ego and a weak trust in a good object (Fairbairn 1952). Grotstein (1981) points out that in a pathological state various symptoms such as loss of appropriate affect and confusion may follow, whereas in the normal infant there is helplessness and relative unintegration. At the paranoid position, Klein described excessive splitting into good and bad of both self and object, with consequent excessive idealization and excessive persecution. She described the excessive projection of bad parts of the self into the object and thus excessive phobic fears or feelings of a paranoid type. Feelings of persecution spiral and escalate, owing to projection into the object and re-introjection of the by now bad objects, producing the need to reproject and so on. It is important to remember, however, that in a footnote in that same 1946 paper, Klein also wrote of how good parts of the self may be projected excessively, with consequent weakening of the ego and feelings of being swallowed up by the excessive goodness and value of the object. This phenomenon is as much a feature of the paranoid position as is the one characterized by projection of the bad part. Constant projection of the good part also produces a vicious circle seen in some very delinquent children and certainly in many psychiatrically depressed children, who may feel incapable of meeting the demands of a needy or damaged object that is felt to be beyond their strength to repair. The blanket of despair seems much more total and all parts of the self and the object seem to be engulfed in it. It is also important to consider that, in some very disturbed and deprived children, the good part and the belief in a good object may not necessarily be projected; it may, instead, be severely underdeveloped.

Splitting

Many authors, both psychoanalytic and psychiatric, have described the states of fragmentation and dissociation to be found in psychosis. Kleinian psychoanalysts have used the close analysis of such states to demonstrate that this seeming randomness may be the product of meaningful processes which involve mental activity and active, emotionally motivated, mentality: dynamic processes such as splitting, disintegration, pathological identification, dismantling, attacks on linking, all of them processes which are seen as designed actively, that is, defensively, destructively or protectively, to perpetuate some state of mind or avoid another (Rosenfeld 1965; Joseph 1987; Meltzer et al. 1975; Bion 1959). Such ideas might seem to be light years away from deficit theory, since they imply defensive activities which interfere with possible integrations in a resistive way. Yet surely mental impoverishment which has become chronic in a young child who should be developing may, whatever the original motivations, result in deficit. Winnicott (1960b), Klein (1946) and Bick (1968) all insisted that states of unintegration should not be confused with disintegration. I would add that anyone who has worked for long with the type of children I have mentioned does not always find evidence of previously acquired integrations.

In other words, it may be necessary to conceive of mental conditions where thoughts remain not dismantled but unmantled; not projected but as yet never introjected; not dissociated but as yet unassociated; not split defensively but as yet not integrated; and where thoughts remain unlinked not because the link has been attacked but because the link has never been forged in the first place. The complication in the live clinical situation is that such situations rarely appear in pure culture and the defensive motives and the defects are invariably mixed. But the distinction is nevertheless crucial for the practising clinician who treats borderline psychotic children: thrusting premature integrations on an already confused child may only confuse him further.

The developmental psychologist Bruner (1968) does not make use of psychoanalytic terms such as splitting, but he does insist that what he calls 'one-trackedness of behaviour' has to be firmly established, and only then, by a series of careful steps, does the baby move to 'two-trackedness'. Bruner describes how babies learn to co-ordinate reaching and grasping, and how, eventually, they become able to maintain intentionality through a sequential series of acts.

He says that the relation between sucking and looking goes through three phases in its growth:

1   The suppression of one by the other: mostly it is looking that suppresses sucking, that is, the neonate cannot suck and look at an interesting object both at the same time. He tends to shut his eyes while sucking. By 3 to 5 weeks he may leave his eyes open while sucking, but if he fixes on or tracks something, sucking stops.
2   By 9–13 weeks there is a new development, a simple succession of sucking and looking, organization by alternation.
3   In the third phase, which he calls place holding, the two acts go on, with one in reduced form that is sufficient for easy resumption, while the other goes into full operation.

Bruner says that usually by 4 months the baby appears to be able to suck and look at once. He explains, however, that although the baby seems to continue sucking while looking, the sucking is not of the suctioning type – the baby continues to mouth the breast but is not drawing in milk. 'By maintaining some feature of an ongoing act in operation while carrying out some other act in parenthesis, one is reminded that the original act is to be resumed.' So the baby is 'tided over the distraction' until he can get back to nutritive sucking (1968: 42). It is rather like putting a finger on the line on the page of a book, while holding a brief conversation.

Bruner's suggestion that suppression precedes alternation and only after alternation is established can place holding be managed, and only with place holding can true co-ordination take place, tells us something important about some of the conditions under which human beings are able to concentrate on ever-widening areas of experience. It throws light on some of my own clinical impressions based on work with ego deficit and thought disorder or, rather, thinking defect. I am reminded of my own belated recognition of how important it was for a patient of mine, Robbie, to learn to forget overexciting ideas and be able to ignore overstimulating sights. He was, for example, easily pulled into a psychotic state where he seemed almost to drown in ecstasy, simply by looking into someone's eyes. When he finally began to want another kind of contact of a more alert but sober kind, one of his first solutions to this problem was to close his eyes, just like Bruner's babies.

Introjection, projection, projective identification

Melanie Klein held to the view that processes of introjection and projection operated from the beginning of life (Spillius 1988). As Paula Heimann put it, 'Life is maintained through the organism's intake of foreign but useful matter and discharge of its own, but harmful matter. Intake and discharge are the most fundamental processes of any living organism' (Heimann 1952). She agreed with Klein that the mind was no exception to this rule, and that, although previous psychoanalysts had accepted that the superego was built up through introjection, it took Klein to point out that so also was the ego. Klein was suggesting that babies, from the start, were capable of learning from experience, absorbing experience, but that they also had some capacity to defend themselves against experience by discharge activities. The model and metaphor was of a digestive system, but it was not, however, a reductive model, and Klein insisted that the baby took in love and understanding at the breast, not simply milk and sensuous satisfaction; many of the experiences described as being taken in or evacuated were seen as mental and emotional.

Klein's work also suggested that it was not enough to look for the discharged aspects of the patient in the repressed and buried unconscious: these missing parts or feelings could sometimes lie much further afield, in someone else's feelings. This phenomenon, called 'projective identification', includes situations where, for example, some people you meet always make you feel intelligent and attractive, while others always make you feel that your slip is showing. Human beings, often quite unknowingly, can evoke very specific and often powerful feelings in other people, and we may do this repetitively in certain systematic ways in order to rid ourselves of unwanted or simply unacknowledged parts of our own personality, or because we genuinely believe a particular feeling or thought or talent could never be ours. A child may indeed have an elder brother who is more intelligent or more academic than she is, but if this fact of her family history has led her to believe that everyone is more intelligent and that she is stupid, she not only may see others as more intelligent (Freud's notion of projection – Freud 1911b), but may be doing something much more active and continuously impoverishing to her own personality than simply having a perception; she may be really allowing or even inviting others to do the thinking for her in situations where she could do it for herself (projective identification as described by Klein 1946).

Bion (1962a), observing in himself the type of projective identification processes mentioned earlier – that is, evoked by the patient – began to notice that sometimes his schizophrenic patients were using these processes neither as a defence nor because the unacknowledged part of the personality was simply unrecognized as theirs, but rather because, in some situations, the patient seemed really to need Bion to carry feelings the patient himself could not bear. Bion suggested that some projective identifications expressed a need to communicate something to someone on a very profound level; he began to see this as related to a fundamental process in normal development, and compared the analyst's 'containment' and 'transformation' of the patient's feelings and thoughts to the primitive but powerful pre-verbal communications that take place between mothers and tiny infants. The mother's capacity for reverie, he wrote, could contain the infant's crises and excitements and transform them into bearable experiences. He suggested that this is normal maternal function, and many analysts have begun to consider this quality of understanding as central to their work with all patients, not only the psychiatrically ill.

This digestive model has offered a rich source for the ways in which experience is assimilated, but it nevertheless need no longer be the only one. Indeed, when the problem has to do with the patient's difficulties in listening, the breast–mouth model may be inadequate. The manner in which experience is assimilated through the visual modality, and also through tactile modes other than oral ones (e.g. the ways in which babies improve upon their capacity to reach and grasp objects in three-dimensional space), may also provide a fertile source for both theory and technique with borderline psychotic children. The fact, for example, that an experience can be assimilated only when it is located in someone else may have more to do with questions of perspective than with questions of projection. Such locating may actually involve the beginnings of an introjective process rather than a projective one. The way in which a patient may or may not be able to follow the therapist's train of thought, or pursue one of his own, may be as analogous to the problem of visual tracking of the trajectory of moving objects as to his response to the flow of milk in his throat.

I have been led to these speculations on the importance of perspective by the observation that some very withdrawn patients may be alerted to a new experience for what seems to be the first time not when it is happening inside them but, rather, when it is seen to be happening inside someone else. Whereas in the past I would have seen this as the result of a projective mechanism, I now think this may be a mistaken formulation. This is because, according to the concept of projection (even the more subtle Kleinian one of projective identification), although the experience is taking place outside the self, it must have originated within the self. That is, the experience projected must have come originally from the patient's self and has been subsequently disowned. Work with very young borderline psychotic children, however, often makes one suspect that the 'projected' part may never have belonged to the personality in the first place, at least not in any solid way. It may need to grow, and this sense of being alive and human may need to be recalled or, in the case of the illest children, called forth (Reid 1990). This need for input from the therapist in order to be recalled to themselves must always be carefully distinguished from the part of the personality which, as it were, can't be bothered to fight for life; the line between apathy consequent on despair and the apathy consequent on hostile indifference or complacent passivity is not an easy one to draw.

Idealization as a development

Here I wish to explore the distinction between processes of idealization used as a defence against persecutory anxiety or depressive pain and processes of idealization which occur as necessary stages of development. Klein and her followers emphasize both functions, but it is interesting that both the Laplanche–Pontalis (1973) and the Hinshelwood (1989) dictionaries of psychoanalytic concepts refer only to Klein's views on the defensive function of idealization. I shall try to demonstrate that the first appearance of ideal objects in the phantasies of chronically depressed children may signal not a resistive or evasive defence against depression, but an important developmental achievement. My interest in this subject was stimulated by a remark of Elizabeth Spillius's concerning the fact that we know little about the growth of idealization.

Laplanche and Pontalis define idealization in the following way: 'Idealisation is the mental process by which the object's qualities and value are elevated to the point of perfection. Identification with the idealised object contributes to the formation . . . [of the] ideal ego and the ego ideal.' They point out that Freud thought that the idealization of the loved object was closely linked to narcissism. Rosenfeld has made a similar link (1964). Klein, in 'Some theoretical conclusions regarding the emotional life of the infant' (1952: 64), states that:

> It is characteristic of the emotions of the very young infant that they are of an extreme and powerful nature. The frustrating bad object is felt to be a terrifying persecutor, the good breast tends to turn into the ideal breast which should fulfil the greedy desire for unlimited, immediate and everlasting gratification. Thus feelings arise about a perfect and inexhaustible breast, always available, always gratifying.

She adds: 'in so far as idealisation is derived from the need to be protected from persecuting objects, it is a method of defence against anxiety.' But she also says:

> While in some ways these defences [splitting and idealization] impede the path of integration, they are essential for the whole development of the ego, for they again and again relieve the

young infant's anxieties. This relative and temporary security is achieved predominantly by the persecuted object being kept apart from the good one.

She goes on to say that object relations are shaped by love and hatred, and permeated on the one hand by persecutory anxiety, on the other by its corollary, which she calls the 'omnipotent reassurance derived from the idealisation of the object' (1952: 70–1). Thus Klein seems at times to be stressing the defensive function in idealization, at others the fact that it is essential for the whole development of the ego. Perhaps a better phrase for the non-defensive essential function of idealization would be 'potent assurance' rather than 'omnipotent reassurance'.

In 'The psychogenesis of manic-depressive states' (1935) Klein again stresses need rather than only defence. She points to two preconditions for the eventual integrations of the depressive position: (1) a strong libidinal relation to part objects and (2) the eventual introjection of the whole object. Again, in the 1940 'Mourning and its relation to manic-depressive states', she says:

> The shaken belief in the good objects disturbs most painfully the process of idealisation, which is an essential intermediate step in mental development. With the young child, the idealised mother is the safeguard against a retaliating or dead mother and against all bad objects and, therefore . . . [perhaps an 'also' would have been better than a 'therefore' to stress the element of need] represents security and life itself.
>
> (1940: 355)

Idealization as a defence: clinical illustration

Alice, a 12-year-old girl, was referred for fairly mild depression, some difficulties with friends, and working slightly below par at school. She had been born with a huge purple birthmark, an angioma, which covered the whole side of her face. It is inoperable while she is still growing but can be operated on when she finishes growing. Very little else can be done for it in the meantime, although her parents have taken her all over the country for various sorts of treatment. In this session she had been waiting for weeks to be given an appointment in London, not her home

city, for laser treatment. The best the treatment could offer was
to create a few tiny white spots in the purple mass. To the outside
observer it would make very little difference, but similar minus-
cule improvements from other treatments seemed to mean a lot
to Alice, and to have kept her hope alive.

The session I wish to mention took place shortly before the
Christmas break, and after several postponements by the laser
clinic in London. Each time the therapist tried gently to help Alice
see that she was feeling frustrated by all the waiting and post-
ponement of her hopes, and by the coming interruption to their
relationship, Alice would momentarily acknowledge it, and then
hasten to speaking about the Alpine skiing she was looking
forward to and how well she remembered it from last year and
how beautiful were the whiteness of the snow and the brightly
shining sun. It seemed to the therapist that, although Alice's
feeling for the purity and beauty of the Alps was genuine, she
was clinging to thoughts about them in order to avoid the painful
dark thwartings of hopes and the irritation with her therapist for
leaving her at such a time.

Alice, I suggest, had a well-developed capacity for idealization
and appreciation of beauty. She took great personal care and
was an attractive girl with lovely shining hair which she arranged
to fall over the discoloured part of her face. She had hope and
strength and determination, and, instead of despairing apathy, a
mild depression due, I think, to a difficulty in feeling permitted
to acknowledge her own rage and impatience to be made to look
normal. In her case, an already developed capacity for idealization was to some extent being used defensively, and she eventually
obtained much relief from interpretations which freed her to feel
the blacker feelings alongside the white. Her depression lifted and
she became more alert and effective at school.

Idealization as a development: clinical illustration

The point I wish to stress is that integration between the bright
and dark side of one's nature and of one's object is possible only
when there is adequate development of both the idealizing
and the persecutory strands. There are quantitative issues here.
Tiny increments in idealization in patients whose capacity for
bright hope is severely underdeveloped should not be exposed to

constant reminders of the very despair and anxiety they are finally managing, not to defend against, but to overcome.

I would like to illustrate the point by describing a very depressed 12-year-old named Ricky, who appeared, almost for the first time, to be conceiving of an ideal object – strangely enough, thanks probably to a television programme.

Ricky had several separations from his mother in the second year of his life. She has had several different violent live-in partners. He is a passive boy who gives the impression of having been clinically depressed for all or most of his life. This session of once-weekly therapy took place after two cancellations, one by him, one by his therapist. When Miss J collected him and called his name, he at first did not respond, and then seemed surprised to see her. In the room he looked into his box and exclaimed, 'Oh good, there's paper in it' and then he muttered a hardly audible thank you. For the first part of the session he remained quite withdrawn, ruling line after line on the page and insisting that these were 'just lines'. When at one point Miss J commented that he might have felt forgotten by her, he said, 'Mm, but you remembered the paper.' She acknowledged his pleasure at this, but as he continued to be in general much less responsive than he had become prior to the two cancellations, she reflected that it seemed very difficult for him to talk to her today, as if he didn't know how or had forgotten how. She suggested that he was telling her that he had lost contact with her and felt out of touch and was now struggling to re-establish a line or link between them. He said, in an off-hand way, that he couldn't really talk while he was drawing, he needed to concentrate. Miss J persisted gently, saying that it seemed especially difficult today after such a long break. He then said, with more enthusiasm, that he thought he would draw a picture of a car he had seen on TV. It was 'an enormous car, ten times the size of this room and the same width. It had everything you could wish for in it, a swimming pool, TV, a telephone so you could phone someone. Also a bath, a fridge, food and a bed. Imagine having something like that all to yourself.' He wished it was his, he 'would never have to leave it for anything. It had everything. You could swim all day in the holidays.'

The therapist then made an interpretation which seemed to see this idealization as a defence. She said that she thought the car stood for her, that he wished he could move in lock, stock and barrel and have her to himself all the time and never have to leave, have a direct line to her (linked with the fact he comes only once a week). He said, 'Mm' and then seemed to deflate. After quite a long pause, she commented on this and asked what he was thinking. He said he was thinking of his aunt. The aunt had split up with her boyfriend and had kicked him out. The boyfriend had arrived at their door asking if they could give him a bed for the night and if they could think of anywhere he could stay. He went on to show that he felt sorry for this man who had been kicked out, and remained deflated for the rest of the session.

This is a moving and disturbing account of the always difficult problem of getting the balance right in working with such disturbed children. I condensed the session considerably, but I hope I have conveyed the degree of devotion with which Miss J persisted in her attempts to understand Ricky's cut-off depression in the first part of the session. It was only after her efforts were rewarded, and his heart lifted, that she lost touch with him. She conveyed great understanding of his depression but not of his sudden burst of happiness. His hopes rose, I think, as her sensitive persistence gave him cause to believe that she really did have him in mind, and indeed probably had had him in mind and not forgotten him over the three-week gap: 'Imagine, something like that all for yourself.' He had, I think, a rush of belief in an object that was available, receptive and somehow full of resources. Looked at from the point of view of mature depressive position development where separateness is acknowledged and objects have to be shared with themselves as well as others, there may be 'defensive' elements in this ideal car. But surely the maternal object has first to be possessed before it can be shared? Dreams have to be dreamed first before they can be shed.

There is a further problem in this session which has to do with the power and reality of transference experiences in the here and now. The therapist took the story of the car to imply a wish for a state which was fundamentally unattainable. She could, instead, have acknowledged that Ricky had actually felt he had just had a surprisingly and unexpectedly good experience – that is, that he was not wishing for, but had in fact found a spacious and available object in her. The idealizing elements in this could then have been dealt with. But overidealization of a state which is fundamentally good or ideal should not be confused with idealization of a state which is fundamentally bad. As it was, I think Ricky felt, like his aunt's boyfriend, kicked out of the new home in his therapist's mind that he had only just found.

In *Listening Perspectives in Psychotherapy*, Hedges (1983: 136) supports Kohut's theory and technique as related to idealized parental imagos. Hedges discusses the weak egos of borderline patients, and says, 'It should be stated that with borderlines therapy is known to be ego-building, but this does not mean that the therapist should or needs to be building anything.' He believes that the analytic work can continue without 'support' or suggestion in direct or guiding forms from the therapist, but that an ego can nonetheless grow. The argument I am pursuing suggests that the process of introjection of an ideal object is a long, slow process. It depends, according to Klein, on whether the child has developed previously a strong positive relationship to part-objects, and therapists should ensure that their interpretative work is tuned to the appropriate level, so that it does not stand in the way of this process.

A clinical example

Some years ago I was treating a little borderline psychotic girl named Judy who suffered from asthma. She had never had an asthma attack in my presence, but one day she came in with a slight shortness of breath and said, in a very anxious voice, that she was having an asthma attack. I tried to show her that she seemed very frightened, as though she thought she was going to die. Her panic and breathing grew worse and I realized that, instead of helping her, my interpretation had increased her anxiety. I thought quickly, and finally said something about the fact that she didn't seem able to tell the difference between a big asthma attack and a little one. It didn't seem to me a particularly profound interpretation, but she said, with surprise and relief, 'Y-e-e-e-s-s' and her breathing improved. I was struck by the fact that a less anxious patient would have heard the implications in my first interpretation (that is, that she would not die), but that this terrified little girl could not. She had an extremely anxious and fragile mother, and I think she heard my first interpretation as though I, too, thought she was about to die. Although she panicked at every parting, however brief, I could never, in the early years, say that she imagined something terrible might happen to one of us during a weekend break: I had to turn the idea around, and talk to her about her difficulty in believing that both of us might make it through and meet again on Monday.

The Analysis of Defence (Sandler and Freud 1985) records a series of discussions with Anna Freud in the 1970s on her book *The Ego and the Mechanisms of Defence*, which was published in 1936. In one of the discussions, Joseph Sandler distinguishes between defences against painful realities and defences towards, which exist in order to gain or maintain a good feeling of security or safety (protective device) (1985: 19). In one of the later meetings, when they are discussing the fact that repression is developmentally a fairly late mechanism of defence, Anna Freud says that projection is used long before repression. Then Sandler says, 'Presumably because repression needs a considerable amount of strength on the part of the ego in order to work'. Anna Freud replies, 'Well, it needs structuralisation of the personality, which isn't there in the beginning.' Then she says, 'If you haven't yet built the house, you can't throw somebody out of it.' Sandler adds, 'Nor keep him locked in the basement' (Sandler and Freud 1985: 238).

Clearly, it is important to think developmentally about these matters: sometimes when the weekend or the summer break is imminent, one can interpret that the patient is really 'somewhere' upset about the coming break, and so is simply repressing it, when in fact he may have successfully split it off and projected it into the therapist. He doesn't feel 'somewhere he is missing her'; he feels she is going to miss him. Depending on the case, the feeling of missing may need to be contained and explored in the therapist for a lengthy period of time, long before the patient may be ready to experience it as belonging to himself (see Joseph 1978: 112). In cases where the house isn't yet built, what may look like an attempt to throw somebody out of the house – to project the suffering infantile part into someone else – may really be a desperate attempt to find any house anywhere.

One is reminded here of Money-Kyrle's stress on the urgent importance of distinguishing between a projective identification motivated by destructive impulses and one motivated by desperation (1977: 463). He thinks analysts ignore this distinction at their peril, and surely in real life mourning is a gradual process. But when analysts and therapists urge patients to face their fears, their yearning, their sadness, long before they have the resources and imagination to do so, they may be asking too much.

Part II

Clinical challenges

Chapter 5

A case of foot and shoe fetishism in a 6-year-old girl

Juliet Hopkins

Fetishism in females is extremely rare. It is therefore of particular interest to attempt to understand its origins in a girl who was only 6 years old when she started psychotherapy. At that time she was psychotic and believed herself to be a boy. The traumatic nature of much of her early experience was revealed through her psychotherapy; information from her mother confirmed and amplified some important aspects of her history. This chapter follows the difficult and dramatic course of treatment and offers an understanding of the girl's presenting symptoms, including her fetishism.

Referral and assessment

Sylvia Z was referred to our clinic at her mother's request when she was just over 6 years old. Mrs Z complained that Sylvia was hyperactive, unmanageable, had many tantrums and wet the bed; she attended a special school for maladjusted children. Sylvia had a younger brother, Enrico, aged 4 years. Her father, Mr Z, had died in a car crash just before her fourth birthday. When the psychiatrist and the social worker met Sylvia they were both convinced from her appearance that she was a boy. Mrs Z explained that Sylvia had insisted on being a boy since her father died. She also mentioned that Sylvia had a very acute sense of smell and that she had a habit of wanting 'to love and kiss' shoes; she would even throw herself on the shoes of strangers to kiss them, salivate on them and bite them. Her interest in shoes had been first evident at 7 months old when she appeared fascinated by her father's shiny shoes. She would draw herself up to them, salivate on them and then suck her thumb. Later, as a toddler, she adopted the habit of taking a pair of her mother's old shoes to bed with her, a habit which still persisted.

Mrs Z was a very defensive young woman who seemed eager for her daughter to have help but reluctant to involve herself. She explained that she could talk to no one about her husband or his death, but in fact did give a brief account of the accident. This occurred just after the family had moved house in order to provide a separate bedroom for the children who until then had slept with their parents. Mr Z had been disqualified from driving so his brother drove him to collect a carpet for the new house. Mr Z's brother lost control of the car, which crashed and Mr Z died instantly, but his brother was uninjured. Mrs Z said she felt only blank at the time and had never cried. Mrs Z described herself as the only child of Jewish parents. Her father died suddenly of a stroke when she was 5 years old and her mother never wept for him. She herself was sent away at once to boarding school. She could remember very little of her mother during her childhood and now seldom saw her. Her mother had remarried while she was away at school and she never got on with her step-father. After leaving school she worked as a secretary until Sylvia was born. Mr Z's family were Italian Catholics who came to England when he was 12 years old. He took many jobs after leaving school, and following his marriage to Mrs Z he studied in the evenings to become an accountant. Mr and Mrs Z met at a concert, and when she became pregnant they decided to get married, despite bitter opposition from both families.

Sylvia was born early and weighed less than 5 pounds. She was placed in an intensive care unit for 16 days and returned home 'feeding three-hourly, taking an hour and a half to feed, and screaming when not feeding'. Mrs Z attempted to breastfeed her for a week but stopped when she herself became ill. She recalled Sylvia's early months as an absolute nightmare. Nothing would pacify Sylvia and Mr Z 'was driven round the bend' by her screaming, which he said prevented him from studying. Mr and Mrs Z had always felt that there was something wrong with Sylvia and this was confirmed for them when a psychologist assessed her at the age of 3 years and announced that she was 18 months retarded. She did not speak fluently or become toilet trained until she was 5 years old.

Enrico was a much easier baby than Sylvia had been and Mr Z became very attached to him in a way he had never been with

Sylvia. Mrs Z was clearly proud of Enrico's development, though two years later, at the age of 6 years, he too was to be deemed maladjusted. Sylvia's initial assessment at our clinic was inconclusive. The psychiatrist was not sure whether to describe her as 'psychotic' or 'borderline'. The psychologist found her completely untestable, but deduced from her speech that she was likely to be potentially of at least low average intelligence. Arrangements were made for Sylvia to have twice-weekly psychotherapy with me and for Mrs Z to meet with Mrs R, an experienced social worker, for twice-weekly casework. More intensive treatment was not feasible.

Impressions of Sylvia during the initial assessment phase

Sylvia started treatment with me when she was 6 years and 4 months old. There were ten sessions before the first holiday break and during this period I gained the following initial impressions.

My first meeting with Sylvia was dominated by my conviction that she must be a boy. Sylvia succeeded in appearing unmistakably male, although in fact her hair length and clothes were equally suitable for either sex and her features were not masculine. It must have been her slightly swaggering gait, aggressive manner and assertive body postures which conveyed her masculinity. When she smiled her whole face lit up and had a radiant quality which was extremely attractive, but she more often looked angry and menacing.

Sylvia was indeed hyperactive. She rarely pursued the same activity for more than a minute and her conversation was as disconnected as her behaviour. Her dark eyes were intensely bright and she was constantly in the grip of extreme and fluctuating emotions. Love, hate, excitement, terror and rage gripped her in rapid succession. The intensity and passion of her ordinary experience is difficult to convey. She seemed helplessly at the mercy of extremely violent feelings which fluctuated arbitrarily, entirely outside her understanding or control.

Sylvia's first two sessions with me differed from subsequent ones in that she was less disorganized and far less violent than she quickly became. She was excitedly concerned with immersing herself in all the paint and glue provided, and made a number of very messy, sticky pictures called, arbitrarily, 'Ghost', 'Dragon', 'Worm', 'Machine in the rain' and 'Peanut butter spreading on bread'. She hit the dragon picture, claiming it had hit her, and she called the dirty paint water 'wee wee', laughing hysterically as she tipped it over my chair. She expressed the fear that I would hit her like her mother did, and at the end she tried to destroy the light in my ceiling by repeatedly hurling a ball at it. The first two sessions were only two days apart, but five days elapsed before the third session. When I went to collect her she looked at me in terror and bolted. There followed a long chase through the clinic until I cornered her under a secretary's desk. When at last she emerged she blurted out angrily, 'Where *were* you? Have you been away on holiday?' In my room she seized her ball and sank her teeth into it. This action ushered in the first of a long series of extremely violent sessions in which Sylvia threatened to kill me and eat me up. She swore profusely, hurled toys and water at me, kicked and spat and flung the furniture about. At other moments she embraced me, spoke affectionately and begged me to visit her home. At all times she was highly involved in relating to me and never withdrew into activities on her own.

In addition to constantly attacking me, usually for no apparent reason, Sylvia was very preoccupied with fantasies of herself being attacked by monsters. Sometimes she begged me to be her friend and to protect her while she imagined the room to be full of attacking monsters. She called the furniture 'Daleks' and seemed convinced that chairs moved across the room to strike her. Her terror was intense and when she kept cowering and ducking as though about to receive a blow from a Dalek or some other monster, I thought she was hallucinating. At other times, instead of enlisting my help against the monsters, she asked me to play the part of a monster and to frighten her, but she could never tolerate this for more than a minute or two.

I first saw Sylvia's fascination with shoes when I found her embracing and slobbering over another patient's boots in the waiting-room. This behaviour often occurred before Sylvia's sessions and Mrs Z did nothing to restrain it although onlookers found it shocking. It happened that I had been wearing a pair of suede boots when I first saw Sylvia, and she was very disappointed about this because she only loved shiny leather.

Mrs Z had not mentioned Sylvia's passionate interest in feet, but this was apparent from the second session when Sylvia excitedly paddled barefoot in water she had spilled, exclaiming, 'Now you can see my foot!' Later she begged me to paddle in the sink with her so she could see our bare feet together. She also wanted me to tickle her toes. Sylvia spent much time paddling in the sink in all the following sessions before the Christmas holiday. It made her deliriously happy to sit with the water up to her knees, often playing with wet pieces of paper which she called meat balls, fish and lettuces. Most frequently she said she was washing and polishing lettuces, throwing out 'the dirty lettuces' and 'the nasty kidney' on to the floor. She sometimes remarked that her feet were cheesy and said that she loved cheesy feet.

Sylvia's feet were important to her as instruments of aggression as well as sources of excited pleasure. When wearing her shoes she liked to stamp items underfoot to destroy them and she kicked me and the furniture often and violently. Sylvia had told me she was a boy soon after we met, when she also remarked that girls were stupid. She did not mind my calling her Sylvia as long as I did not refer to her as 'she' or 'her'.

Sylvia's excitement about paddling at the sink increased from session to session. She wanted to flood the whole room so that it would be a swimming pool which she could wee into. At the height of her excitement she stood on top of the sink, pulled down her jeans and pants, and with her hands indicated the invisible arc of urine she supposed to be spurting forth to soak me. I said she really believed she was weeing from a big willy and Sylvia agreed as though she were convinced of it. Next session she announced she was a man diver who would dive into my pool and she managed to take off her clothes and stand naked on the window-sill 'so everyone can see me do it'. All these activities were carried out with tremendous excitement and laughter.

In a later session Sylvia showed some doubts about being a boy. Revealing her pink underpants, she remarked, 'Boys *do* wear these, don't they?' And in the same session she also referred to herself as 'her'. When I commented on her doubts about being a boy she confirmed them by squatting and urinating on the floor behind a chair 'to serve you right', in totally different style from the earlier manic deluded moment when she had indicated that she was urinating from a penis. Sylvia had inadvertently referred to herself as 'her' when we were talking about how she had attacked me in the waiting-room. Sylvia explained, 'That was the other Sylvia who hit you, not me. I socked *her* in the eye.' She had previously insisted that there were two Mrs Hopkins – a horrid one in the waiting-room and a nice one in my room. On many occasions she looked at me quizzically as though bewildered about who I was, and asked, 'Where's the other Mrs Hopkins gone?' I thought she was the victim of an extreme form of defensive splitting which she used principally to deal with anxieties about my return after separation. Mrs Z reported that Sylvia had become intensely attached to me, spoke of me continuously at home and could not wait for her sessions. However, by the time I saw her, Sylvia could only greet me with terror and rage, attacking me by hurling toys or running away to hide. I had become the horrible Mrs Hopkins of the waiting-room. The end of each session was also unbearable for her. She clung to me or tried to carry on playing until I had to steer her through the door. Then she began at once to scream for her mother and kept this up until they were reunited.

Sylvia's speech was fluent and ranged from the poetic to the obscene. She spoke of inanimate objects as though they were alive, for example, 'The door won't let me open it', or 'I must wake up my sleepy socks – they're falling down'. Her endless fantasies about monsters and space were sometimes delightfully expressed: 'Be a moon, and we'll have star teas', or 'Inside this space is the darkness of the dream monsters'. Her use of 'I' and 'you' was clear and accurate. When she was angry she swore with a range of obscenities which she was unlikely to have picked up from other children.

Therapeutic approach

During this early period of Sylvia's treatment I struggled to impose some order on her chaos and on my own confusion by simply trying to describe what was happening and by naming the emotions which she was experiencing with me. When I had identified her feelings I tried to link them with the few sequences I understood, for example her anger because she had to wait for me and her terror that I would retaliate whenever she was angry. I emphasized that I was *one* person whom she sometimes loved and sometimes hated and feared, and that there were not two Mrs Hopkins or two Sylvias either. I spoke of her evident bewilderment about whether I and other grown-ups were friends or enemies, whether we would protect her or kill her, and I indicated how she tried to allay her fears that I would attack her unpredictably by actively trying to provoke an attack under her control.

In her quieter moments Sylvia clearly welcomed understanding and found some of my comments meaningful.

Sylvia's enormous erotic excitement about feet, shoes and willies made me very cautious about giving interpretations in sexual terms because of the risk of provoking uncontrollable excitement and exhibitionism. Behind her manifest excitement about sexual matters I sensed an extreme anxiety and this reinforced my caution about interpreting sexual themes, both at this phase and throughout the treatment.

As far as Sylvia's actual sex was concerned, in early treatment I acknowledged that she often needed to believe she was a boy or a man with a willy so she could excite me and feel as close to me as being married. However, I told her that I could see that she really knew she was a girl. I made no comments about Sylvia's excited interest in feet, but I linked her voracious attacks on shiny shoes in the waiting-room with her feelings about my absence, the pain of waiting to embrace me and the fear both of my failure to return and of my return to attack her. In order not to excite her interest in my shoes I decided always to wear the same pair of suede boots when I saw her, and I did this throughout the first year of her treatment.

During this first phase of work with Sylvia I did not try to interpret any of her material in relation to her past and present experiences outside the clinic. It seemed essential to reduce her most intense anxieties about seeing me before we could think about the origins of her preoccupations.

Possible diagnosis: traumatic psychosis

After this initial phase of therapy I found myself wondering whether Sylvia had been traumatized by violent treatment. On reflection, this impression seemed to be based on the following lines of evidence which I report in some detail, as the importance of trauma in psychotic and borderline conditions may sometimes be overlooked.

First my countertransference. After each session Sylvia left me feeling emotionally bruised, betrayed and bewildered by the constantly reiterated shocks of her sudden switches from affectionate overtures to violent assaults. I thought my experience with her might well reflect experiences which she herself had suffered. Second, my work with three neurotic child patients who had had similarly intense, though more intellectual, preoccupations with monsters had led me to recognize that such preoccupations commonly represent not just the child's own monstrous feelings, but also the adults who were responsible for arousing these feelings. Analysis of the monsters in the three cases mentioned revealed that they disguised, respectively, a history of physical abuse by the mother, a homosexual assault, and early hospitalization experiences (Hopkins 1977). In each case the monsters represented a compromise between the child's fear of *real* aggressive attacks and fears related to his own aggressive impulses.

Sylvia had not yet mentioned her father but the nature of her monsters and her response to my absences made me suppose she had experienced him as a terrifying person who would return to avenge his death. She appeared to have dealt with his loss by identifying with him, and it seemed probable that this identification, an identification with the aggressor, had begun before he died, in response to her fear of him.

Another suggestive aspect of Sylvia's material was her use of her craziness to camouflage reality. At moments when she was relatively sane she would suddenly escape into distracting psychotic fantasies if I mentioned an aspect of reality she didn't like, such as the coming holiday. It seemed she might be unconsciously exploiting her madness as a camouflage to hide some unacceptable truths. At this stage her capacity for camouflage effectively confused me and prevented me from realizing that her terror was a terror for her life, and not a psychotic fear of personal annihilation or disintegration (Rosenfeld 1975).

Several factors corroborate my impression that Sylvia had been the victim of physical violence. The literature on abused children offers some external support (Delozier 1982). Sylvia was hyperalert. Her need to be constantly involved with me had a monitoring quality and she never turned her back. Later in treatment when she no longer defensively split me into two Mrs Hopkins, she came to manifest an acute approach–avoidance conflict on first meeting me which is characteristic of abused children. Stroh's (1974) data on seven children diagnosed as suffering from traumatic psychosis provide an essentially similar diagnostic picture. All of these children suffered from panic rages and extreme contradictory behaviour in which they violently attacked the people they loved, eliciting counter-aggression which repeatedly re-created their early experiences. Finally, Sylvia's excited, erotic behaviour towards feet and shoes merits description as fetishism, a condition which implicates a variety of physical and sexual trauma in its development (Greenacre 1979; Stoller 1975), but which has not previously been reported in a child with a traumatic psychosis.

When giving her account of Sylvia's early history, Mrs Z had made no mention of family violence. In fact, she had told more in this first interview than she was to reveal for a very long time to come. Although she met twice weekly with Mrs R, she quickly became extremely withdrawn and often spent whole sessions in angry or remote silence. She was too threatened by questions to answer any, so many details of Sylvia's history had to remain unknown. However, in her own time she gradually amplified the initial outline she had given with important material to be reported later. But, meanwhile, it was to be Sylvia herself who conveyed information about some of her early experiences through her play and behaviour in her sessions with me.

Trauma reconstruction and exorcism: sessions 11–31

After Christmas Sylvia enabled me to reconstruct some of her experiences before her father died, two and a half years previously. She increasingly demanded that I should act the part of terrifying monsters who pursued her with roars and threatened to eat her up. 'Be a Dalek', 'Be a carpet monster' (draped in a carpet), or 'Be a light-switch monster', she said. By this means I thought she was trying to localize and control her terrors of being attacked, but it was never wholly successful for she often screamed out in terror that a chair, a light or an unseen monster was attacking her.

I first interpreted one of her dramas as an attempt to communicate the past in a session when she told me, 'Be a cross dream!' She made herself a bed and hid under the blanket. 'Roar!' she shouted. When I did, she asked, 'Are you a *real* mummy? Are you a daddy too?' 'Yes,' I said. 'Speak Italian then!' she replied. 'I'm "Never Mind Boy" in bed. I'm not Sylvia. Sylvia was too frightened.' I said she was trying to remember what it was like when she was little and her mummy and daddy had had terrible roaring rows in Italian and she had been too frightened to bear it. 'Go tap, tap with your feet,' said Sylvia urgently. I had to stamp with a regular rhythm. I asked, 'Did mummy and daddy go tap,

tap with their feet?' Sylvia replied, '*Not* with their bottoms, silly. With their *feet*.'

This was the first occasion on which Sylvia revealed her confusion between feet and genitals, and also indicated how she had dealt with night terrors about parental violence and sexuality by imagining herself to be a boy. She was moved by my reconstruction and wanted me to tell her more about what had happened in the past. During part of each session she would enact a drama in a particularly urgent manner which I understood as a request for me to reconstruct past events, which were at first more rows between her fighting parents. Sylvia now claimed to remember their fights. 'Dad beat my mummy up,' she said with conviction.

Soon Sylvia voiced more memories of her own. One session when she asked me to 'be a fierce daddy monster and frighten me very much', I said I thought she was trying to remember how she had been frightened of her own fierce daddy. Sylvia suddenly looked at me with great amazement and said, 'My dad broke up our house! It was another house. He threw all the furniture.' She was perplexed about where this event had happened and I told her I knew she had lived with her dad in a different house which her family left just before he died. Sylvia replied in a disconnected and cheerful way, 'You haven't seen my feet for a long time,' and she proceeded to paddle in the sink. She interrupted this activity to say, 'Be my friendly dad in my house. Come and listen to my record. Get in my bed.' When I came close to her she suddenly changed from friendliness to panic. 'My dad was in my bed. A terrible dream! A giant crane was rising up! And now a screwdriver is coming!' Sylvia held out her arms to protect her abdomen. 'The crane killed me with a sharp knife,' she concluded with a shudder. I said she might be trying to remember being terrified of dad's giant willy. Sylvia didn't appear to listen. She asked brightly, 'What is paper made of?' and returned to washing her paper lettuces.

Sylvia's vivid recollection of her father throwing furniture helped me to understand her terrors of flying Dalek furniture and her own need to overturn and fling the furniture herself. She quickly responded to interpretation about her wish to throw furniture in order to terrify me so I would know how she had felt when her father did it. She lost her terror of being attacked by furniture and also stopped throwing it.

In her role of 'Never Mind Boy', Sylvia began to think increasingly about the past. Just as her recollection of her father throwing furniture had laid the Dalek monsters to rest, so her recollection that her father had died in a car accident, collecting a carpet, led to the disappearance of her need to make me attack her dressed as a 'carpet monster' (always pronounced by her as 'car-pit'). Sylvia's attacks on the lights in my room and her terror of the 'light-switch monster' seemed related to her intense fear of the dark and her almost equal fear of turning on the light to reveal her monster parents fighting or banging their feet together. Discussion of these fears stopped Sylvia's attacks on the lights, and the light-switch monster also disappeared.

Soon after this Mrs Z told Mrs R that Sylvia had asked her about the old house and Mrs Z had taken her to see it. Whether or not at this time Mrs Z and Sylvia were also able to share memories of Mr Z's violence we do not know, since a whole year was to elapse before Mrs Z at last confirmed Sylvia's memories by confessing to Mrs R that her husband had thrown furniture in his rages and had broken the arms off the chairs. She said he had also beaten Sylvia frequently and had thrown her across the room. When Sylvia was a screaming baby he had 'kicked' both mother and daughter out of the house 'or else he would have killed Sylvia'. His violence outside the home had led him into trouble with the police. As for Sylvia's possible indication of some sexual advance from her father, no external confirmation was ever forthcoming. I return to this subject later.

After reconstructing some of the events which seemed to have contributed to her intense terrors of monsters, Sylvia began to bring happier memories about her father. She liked to sit on top of my cupboard because it was just like 'riding on my daddy's back'. She told me with delight how she could now remember going to the park with her daddy and paddling with him in the pool. She began to ask me to 'be a friendly daddy' while she was 'Never Mind Boy' and we went to the park together. Sylvia was now in touch with her love for her friendly father as well as her hatred and fear of her fierce and angry father. At this stage I seemed to represent in turn both aspects of her father, and Sylvia had not yet accepted the reality of his loss.

Sylvia continued to express a persistent desire to see and to smell 'your lovely white feet'. When I told her of the coming Easter holiday she told me how she dreamed of going away with me, taking off my shoes and socks and paddling with me at the seaside. She was very aware of being rejected by me and was acutely jealous of my husband who she was sure would paddle with me. This holiday was to confront her with the reality of losing me and after it she was able to acknowledge the loss of her father.

By the time that Easter came, Mrs Z reported great improvements. Sylvia had stopped having violent tantrums and now talked about what angered her. She had become much more manageable and no longer made advances to strangers' shoes. She had also stopped bed-wetting and did not insist she was a boy, though she was still reluctant to admit to being a girl. At school her teacher reported that she had at last begun to learn.

At the clinic Sylvia no longer supposed that there were two Mrs Hopkins and her behaviour in the waiting-room and corridor had become much more controlled. She was still preoccupied with monsters but no longer possessed by them. After Easter Mrs R and I both independently observed how Sylvia had lost that radiant quality of beauty which she possessed when she started treatment. A beautiful boy was changing into a plain little girl. The terror and the masculinity had gone and with them the radiance too. I felt as though something comparable to exorcism had happened and I wondered what had been instrumental in achieving this change. It was my impression that it was Sylvia's recall of past traumatic events, facilitated by my reconstruction, which had alleviated her most florid psychotic symptoms. She became dispossessed of a primitive identification with her father, which had been split into an idealized omnipotent aspect which she embodied and a terrifying persecutory one which she attributed to monsters. Instead of being possessed by images of her father she became able to know about him.

The ready availability of Sylvia's memories had surprised me. Evidently the traumatic events which she recalled must have been registered cognitively by her at the time of their occurrence. My reconstruction effectively gave her permission, in a safe setting, to recall and to share what she already knew. The analytic literature (Bowlby 1979; Khan 1972; Rosen 1955; Tonnesmann 1980) suggests that the therapist's ability to construct external events is of particular importance when the patient has taken psychotic flight from reality or when important adults in the patient's life have put a taboo on knowing. In both these conditions, which applied to Sylvia, the therapist risks colluding with the patient's defences if he treats the traumatic events only as fantasies. He may also risk repeating the behaviour of the original traumatogenic adult, for, as Balint (1969) points out, it is common for an adult who has traumatized a child to behave afterwards as though nothing had happened and as though the child had simply imagined it.

In Sylvia's case the shared acknowledgement of terrifying events in her past provided a key to her plight for both of us. Although we could never know the exact nature of her past experience, we had both gained a cognitive framework in which to organize evidence. Sylvia now became sufficiently in touch with reality to learn in school. In treatment she had increasing periods of quiet and thoughtful behaviour when she drew pictures and talked about them. After Easter she moved on to acknowledge further aspects of reality: her lack of a penis and the loss of her father. She grew openly depressed and cried recurrently as she genuinely mourned the dad she had loved as well as feared and hated. However, despite all these positive developments, Sylvia could still suddenly become crazy and chaotic. Her progress at this stage must not be exaggerated. Her moods continued to change arbitrarily and although she no longer fought me as though fighting for her life she remained extremely aggressive.

Fetishism, incest and revenge

In the second year of treatment Sylvia continued to make educational progress and behaved well at school. She also gave up her fetishism and began to become aware of some of her emotional problems. She felt herself to be seriously damaged and she feared going mad. This development was associated with less desirable changes. Sylvia felt both suicidal and vengeful and she revelled in punishing and humiliating both me and her mother. I will now describe and comment on these developments and their relationship to the possibility that Sylvia had been the victim of incest.

First, it should be mentioned that, in addition to using shoes and feet as fetish objects, Sylvia had another fetish which she used exclusively for sexual purposes. This was a tobacco tin which she always used when she masturbated. It had been given to her by 'Sir', her class teacher, and it contained 'magic words', Sylvia's name for flash-cards used for reading practice. Sylvia called masturbation 'swimming on my tin'. She lay happily on her stomach under my desk with her head on two cushions and her genitals pressed against the tin, rhythmically moving her hips. Ideally she liked me to 'tap-tap' with my feet while she did this.

Cases of female fetishism are extremely rare in the psychoanalytic literature, but Sylvia's form of masturbation was reminiscent of that used by an adult female patient (Zavitzianos 1971) who could only masturbate to orgasm if she employed a fetish symbolizing her father's penis. However, Sylvia's fetish comprising Sir's magic words in a tin seemed to symbolize the penis in the vagina, while Sylvia 'swimming' under my desk could be interpreted to represent father in intercourse with her mother. By adding the rhythmic noise of my feet she reproduced her version of their sexual act, with herself as a participant and not as an excluded observer.

Sylvia gradually gave up masturbating in sessions and I thought this was related to her growing awareness of being a girl. This new awareness greatly increased her envy and jealousy of Enrico, and Mrs Z reported that she had become most intolerant of him at home. She expressed the wish to bite his willy to bits and she tried to steal his masculinity by borrowing his underpants, his cowboy costume and his tie, which she often wore during sessions. His clothes restored her self-esteem and made her confident of winning my affection. Without them, at times when she accepted being a girl, she was liable to complain that I didn't love her at all. It had been known from the start of treatment that Mr Z had loved Enrico much more than Sylvia. Mrs Z now confessed that she had convinced herself when pregnant that Sylvia would be a boy and had bought only boys' clothes for her. When she gave birth to a girl she was glad that the baby was taken into special care and that she could leave the hospital without her.

Sylvia's fascination with footwear slowly diminished, for reasons which I did not understand, and I began to be able to wear a restricted variety of shoes without exciting her. However, her desire to see and smell my feet and to paddle with me remained at high pitch. It only abated after more work was done on its meaning. This work was facilitated by information given by Mrs Z. I had often wondered what part Sylvia's parents might have played in her choice of fetishes. I had become convinced that she had been overexcited by someone tickling her feet and pretending to eat her toes when she was little. I also thought it likely that she had slept at the foot of her parents' bed so that she had seen their feet move in intercourse.

Mrs Z now told Mrs R that her husband had often encouraged Sylvia to play with his bare feet. In particular she remembered Sylvia as a toddler putting marbles between his toes. Mrs Z also mentioned that he always slept naked and walked about the house naked too. When Sylvia was about 2 years old she had screamed at the prospect of having a bath and would only take a bath sitting on her father's lap, which she regularly used to do.

On the next occasion when Sylvia played at paddling with daddy I asked her if she remembered paddling with him in the bath. 'Oh yes!' said Sylvia ecstatically, 'with his nice friendly willy.' Then immediately she enacted a terrified girl in a park, attacked by a nasty man with a crocodile who broke into the park through a hole. He was shot by a bow and arrow. I said she seemed to have two sorts of memories about daddy's willy in the bath. Sometimes it had seemed nice and friendly, but sometimes she had felt it was fierce like a crocodile and would break into her hole and hurt her. It was safer to be a boy with a bow-and-arrow willy, like 'Never Mind Boy', than a girl with a hole who could be hurt.

If Sylvia had been so frightened of her father's penis, why had she found it reassuring to bath on his lap when she was about 2 years old? Did she feel safe from assault by seeing his penis between her legs and imagining that this frightening organ was her own? Or did the sight of her own and her father's feet in the water help to reassure her that genital differences did not exist? Such relevant material as Sylvia brought before the next holiday confirmed her focus on feet as a displacement from genital differences. It also suggested that Sylvia had enjoyed sexual stimulation in the bath, for she asked me to tickle her genitals while pretending I was her daddy bathing her.

The episode of the break into the park through a hole led to my first mention of Sylvia's vagina. She soon brought much more material which could be understood in terms of her having a vulnerable hole which could be violated by her father's penis. For example, she brought three rubber crocodile monsters to visit her in her bed where she greeted them with an orgy of kissing and sucking before she screamed that they were attacking her. Then she pulled down her pants to show me her genitals and anus, in a manner intended to be very offensive. 'See! That's my blood!' she said. I spoke of her need to convey to me the horrifying shock that she felt when she imagined that her body holes were wounds made by an attacking willy. At this point Sylvia's dominating identification with her father had given way to a more primitive identification with her wounded mother.

Episodes like this were a reminder of the possibility that Sylvia had herself experienced genital assaults or acts like fellatio. Since her early dramatization of attack by crane and screwdriver, which was repeated on three occasions, other suggestive evidence of abuse had come mainly from Sylvia's provocative habit of copious spitting. When Sylvia spat at me she aimed mainly for my mouth and was triumphant when she hit it. She called her spitting 'being sick' and spoke of spitting out poison and of spitting at me to kill me. At first I thought Sylvia's confusion of 'spit' and 'sick' might arise from observations of her baby brother 'spitting' up milk or simply from her fantasy. However, Sylvia told me, 'Willies are sick' and 'I'm sicking out white like a willy'. Perhaps Sylvia had experienced ejaculation in her mouth which had made her feel sick, but I never felt sure enough to suggest it. Certainly Sylvia spat most at times when she was dominated by identification with her father, and as this identification diminished, so did the spitting.

Did Sylvia experience sexual advances from her father or could such mechanisms as identification with her mother and erotization account for her interpretation of violent sexual assaults being directed against herself? Greenacre (1953; 1968) has described how in the pre-fetishist there is a prolongation of the early state of primary identification with the mother, on account of an insecure, unstable body image which impedes separation of the 'I' from the 'other'. In addition to such an identification, Sylvia may have erotized the many beatings she is known to have received from her father, for it is believed that pain and distress in infancy always arouse both sexual and aggressive drives (Freud 1924; Greenacre 1968).

Although identification and erotization may help to explain Sylvia's feelings of having been sexually assaulted, it should also be added that Mrs Z with great reluctance admitted to Mrs R that as a child she herself had been sexually abused by her step-father; she would not give details. It is known that some mothers who were sexually abused in childhood condone the sexual abuse of their own daughters. Certainly Mrs Z had not protected Sylvia from viewing full details of sexual intercourse, which is likely to have been very violent on occasion. With hindsight, now that I am familiar with recent evidence on child sex abuse (e.g. Renvoize 1982), I think it is very likely that Sylvia had not only witnessed violent intercourse, but had played with her father's penis in the bath and had experienced fellatio and possibly even attempts at penetration. She had apparently enjoyed the sex play and in association with this she played games in treatment in which she was a princess who proudly controlled the erections of a crane (a chair-leg under a blanket). However, fellatio seemed to have been associated not only with excitement but with extreme anxiety, humiliation and disgust, while the risk of penetration was clearly terrifying.

During Sylvia's treatment I lacked confidence to reconstruct her sexual activities with her father explicitly, but I described the themes of sex play, fellatio and penetration in terms of her wishes and fears, and also related them to her difficulty in distinguishing what she had seen happening to her mother from what she had supposed was happening to herself. Following this work Sylvia lost interest in my feet, and her mother reported a similar improvement at home.

It seemed to me that Sylvia's foot fetishism, like her masturbatory fetishism, had represented a re-creation of sexual acts. Sylvia's first aim was to see, smell, suck and salivate over a pair of feet (or shoes), thus reproducing the act of fellatio, displaced from penis to feet. Her second, and more important, aim was to paddle with the feet so that there were two pairs of feet together. When Sylvia had bathed with her father at the age of 2 she may have felt that their feet together reproduced the sexual union of the parental couple. The similarity of their feet allowed Sylvia to disavow their sexual differences, while simultaneously Sylvia seems to have been in some ways aware of her father's 'friendly willy', either as a possession or as a source of stimulation. Freud (1938) describes how the split in the ego of fetishists enables them to maintain two such contradictory attitudes at once. Splitting allows them to disavow their perception of a woman's lack of a penis while simultaneously recognizing its absence and experiencing castration anxiety. Freud's fetishistic patients were all men. In Sylvia's case it seemed that she had disavowed sexual differences and armed herself with the fantasy of possessing a penis in order to protect herself from an underlying fear of violation. However, in so far as she still actually believed that she possessed a penis, she may have been liable to castration anxiety. Greenacre (1979) claims that symptoms of fetishism only develop in females in whom the illusionary phallus has gained such strength as to approach the delusional. Sylvia certainly had a major delusion of this kind when treatment started, and although by this stage she had already recognized her lack of a penis and had wept about it, it is possible that the delusion may still have persisted in the enclave of her fetishism. However, it could also be possible that in females fetishism might arise in response to the terror of violation, and that the illusionary phallus and castration anxiety are secondary to this fear.

At the same time as Sylvia lost her excited interest in feet she became conscious of a pervasive sense of bodily damage. For example, she identified closely with 'a squashed rabbit bleeding from its bottom' and a hedgehog alleged to be torn apart and eaten by a Turkish family. She dramatized herself as the victim of terrifying forces which had destroyed her bodily integrity. She also became aware of being psychologically damaged and expressed the fear that she would grow up crazy.

Sylvia had been reasonably well behaved at the clinic for some time, but now when she had an audience she delighted in displaying her disturbance. She aimed deliberately to shock people and show them she was damaged. She spat on other patients and shouted obscenities, 'So they think I'm mad' and 'So they'll know it's all your fault', '*You* broke me', 'You tore me apart'. She repeatedly threatened to throw herself down the stairwell, 'so everyone will know how horrid you've been', and at home she talked of strangling herself. She drew obscene pictures of me and attacked me with her faeces. She revelled in humiliating me and was revengeful and triumphant. In these moods, which mercifully never dominated treatment, her intense hatred had a new and vengeful quality and I found her loathsome.

Although Sylvia now felt seriously damaged, she made no intellectual connection between this and her traumatic history. Perhaps it was too distressing to think that her loved parents were responsible. The earliest and most serious trauma she had suffered was probably her mother's failure to protect and comfort her. Now that I had helped to remove the protection of her fetishism, Sylvia took revenge on me.

These detrimental changes baffled me until I understood them in Stoller's terms (1975). He describes fetishization as an act of cruelty whose unconscious aim is to seek revenge on the original loved traumatizing object, to desecrate it and humiliate it. The accompanying excitement is not due to voluptuous sensations so much as to 'a rapid vibration between the fear of trauma and the hope of triumph'. The trauma feared is the repetition of a childhood event, sensed as life-threatening, and the triumph is the fantasy of revenge on the original loved traumatizing object. When Sylvia ceased to express these complex feelings through her fetishism, it seems that they became expressed instead in object relationships. The triumph of the fetishistic re-enactment of traumatic sexual scenes gave way to acknowledgement of a sense of trauma and a desire for revenge.

Casework with Mrs Z

Mrs Z now insisted on stopping treatment in order to take a job, while the psychologist attached to Sylvia's school thought Sylvia was ready to transfer to a school for normal children. Plans had to be made to end treatment after two years of work.

Mrs R had had a very difficult time working with Mrs Z, who had remained extremely resistant throughout. However, it had been possible, to a limited extent, to help her to mourn her husband and to become able to speak about him with her children. Work had also been done on her overidentification with Sylvia, expressed by Mrs Z as being like one person going into another and dissolving them. Mrs Z's parents had intended that she herself should have been a boy, so her identification with her own unwanted girl baby dated from Sylvia's birth. Mrs R's work with Mrs Z was crucial to the success of Sylvia's treatment, for she managed to maintain her co-operation in spite of her recurrent threats to break off treatment, and also enabled her to make changes which benefited Sylvia. Sylvia must have been further helped by having the same man teacher throughout her treatment, for 'Sir' was a kindly father-figure whom Sylvia loved.

Treatment was nearly over before Mrs Z admitted how 'utterly brutal' her own relationship to Sylvia had always been and continued to be. Sylvia was certainly extraordinarily provocative but Mrs Z's collusion with this was most unfortunate. It seemed that Mrs Z needed to continue a violent relationship with Sylvia, although she also loved her and wanted to help her. It had taken two years of patient work with this defensive mother to reveal the extent of Sylvia's rejection from birth and of both parents' murderous feelings towards her. Sylvia's inability to acknowledge that it was her parents who had threatened her life, and her misattribution (Bowlby 1973) of this threat to monsters, may have been partly due to the overwhelming terror associated with the realization that both her parents had often wished her dead.

At the end of treatment Mrs Z also revealed that her step-father, who had sexually abused her, had been a shoe-fetishist. This perversion can scarcely have been a complete coincidence, and it may explain the great importance which Mrs Z had attached to Sylvia's first display of interest in her father's shiny shoes. Dickes (1978) has described how parental reactions influence the development of their children's fetishism. As a rejected baby on the floor Sylvia may have been first attracted to shiny shoes as a substitute for faces with their shiny eyes, but her later passion for shoes seemed to stem from their relationship to feet and from the fact that shoes could be possessed, taken to bed, bitten and sucked without retaliation.

Termination

During the last term of her treatment Sylvia always wore skirts, which she now preferred to jeans. She maintained a rigid split between her loving self which appreciated and depended on me, and her damaged and revengeful self which continued to delight in fierce attacks. She still switched from one self to the other without apparent reason or awareness. The main work that was done was on the conflict she experienced between 'wrapping herself inside her mother' and separating from her, and the relationship of this theme to her sexual identity, which was still very confused. She began to think more about me as a separate person with a home and family of my own, from which she felt painfully excluded. Sylvia had been very upset by the decision to end her treatment. In spite of her distress she kept the final date constantly in mind and told me with feeling how much she would miss me. At the end she embraced me in tears and said, 'I cannot bear to say goodbye.'

Follow-up

Sixteen months after treatment ended, when she was nearly 10 years old, Sylvia came to see me again at her own request. She asked me to arrange treatment for herself and for Enrico and was angry when I explained that Mrs Z could not manage to bring them at present. She drew obscene pictures of me to express her rage, but followed them with 'a lovely picture' of me to make amends. This was the first reparative gesture I had ever seen her make.

Mrs Z reported that Sylvia had maintained her gains and there had been no recurrence of her fetishism. She was coping adequately in her normal school where her behaviour was good, but she took it out on her mother after school and was often very difficult to manage. She was growing in independence and successfully performed errands on her own. Despite her great improvements Sylvia remains a borderline child who is likely to encounter very serious problems at adolescence, such as psychosis, promiscuity or attempted suicide.

Acknowledgement

Copyright © Institute of Psychoanalysis

I would like to acknowledge Dr John Bowlby's helpful comments on the manuscript.

Chapter 6

From the 'Drunken boat' to the 'Chinese junk'

The treatment of an 8-year-old boy with severe ego impairment

Beatrice Smith

> As I was floating down unconcerned rivers,
> I no longer felt myself steered by the haulers:
> Gaudy redskins had taken them for targets,
> Nailing them naked to coloured stakes.
> > Translated from Arthur Rimbaud's
> > 'Le Bateau ivre' by Oliver Bernard
> > (Penguin Classics, 1997)

How best could I describe the initial feeling Kim gave me when I met him? Since then, many metaphors have come to mind, which in a concrete way he has confirmed in the many balsa-wood models he has produced in his sessions, from a lost boat, ill assembled, on the verge of sinking but with multiple cannons ready to shoot, to a graceful Chinese junk.

In psychodynamic terms, Kim struck me as having an ego deficiency, unable to process his thoughts or harness his drives, losing grip on reality at times of acute anxiety. In his object relationships, he oscillated unpredictably between fusion with, and rejection of, his primary objects.

I will review the first two years of intensive psychoanalytic psychotherapy with this 8-year-old boy. I will illustrate how, through our transference–countertransference relationship, he was enabled gradually to strengthen his ego and begin to internalize whole, separate and benevolent-enough objects. This led to his development of a more unified and stable identity as well as a growing capacity to symbolize.

I hope that this chapter will also give an idea of the countertransferential aspects of therapist's work in all its vicissitudes: her pain, but also her excitement at a child's new abilities to work analytically.

Background

Kim was referred, aged 8, by his school, who were extremely concerned about this 'most unusual child'. Their report described a child unable to follow normal curriculum activities, who would spend most of the time drawing monsters, or attacking other children or teachers. He was also sexually provocative, asking other children to suck his penis or acting out sexual intercourse with them. He had no friends and was bullied. Mother supported the referral, as she found him uncontainable and was desperate for help.

Kim was an only child who lived with his mother. When she was five months pregnant, she left his father and contact between them stopped totally when Kim was 2. We know very little about father, as mother was very reluctant to open up on the matter. She reported that Kim was always a poor sleeper but that night terrors appeared from the age of 2. Interestingly, these terrors abated, according to mother, when he started to draw – these were always drawings of enormous faces. At the time of referral he continued to have some nightmares in which he would scream and lash out in his sleep. He also, occasionally, wet his bed.

When he was around 3, his very sparse language, inability to relate or play and his finger games (he displayed repetitive, rhythmical movements of his fingers) led to some suspicion of autism. No assessment ensued. At 5, he was sexually abused by a handicapped adolescent boy (the son of a friend of his mother), having to perform fellatio, after which he showed more sexualized behaviour at school. No further details about the abuse were given.

Kim had never been able to settle into school. He had always been bullied and had displayed a lot of violence himself. During the assessment, mother reported some dramatic scenes between them in public. They would hit one another, have violent rows in the street and not be able to contain themselves.

At the diagnostic assessment some of his responses to the Rorschach had a psychotic quality. They revealed a frail hold on reality and how his ability to organize his thought processes could decline under the impact of primitive fantasies; on card seven (mother card), he said, 'Two bunnies kissing . . . They're having sex, there's their body. They're ripping themselves, they're ripping their bodies up.' He was also found to have difficulties in recognizing and regulating his feelings and excitement. His frustration tolerance was low, which interfered with his cognitive capacities.

In all, he gave the impression of a disturbed child, whose shifting object relationships, fragile ego, lack of anxiety signal and poor reality testing suggested a borderline diagnosis. The sexual abuse must have added to his confusion and perception of sexual intercourse as a physical attack, raising acute, overwhelming death anxiety.

Early phase of treatment: first impressions of Kim's psychological strengths and weaknesses

Very early on in his therapy, as early as in his first session, I could detect very distinct signs of Kim's pathology but I could also pick up on certain ego strengths that would help in our work. Both his pathology and his strengths guided me in my work and the pace of my work.

In our initial meeting Kim was extremely anxious, looking very concerned about what sort of a person I was and what I was up to. I intuitively did not verbalize this fear as I sensed it would have stirred up his panic to uncontainable levels. Instead, I chose to address the more general uneasiness about being in this unfamiliar place with an unknown person. To relieve what I felt was some additional anxiety about my obvious foreign accent I answered his question about my age and country of origin. He proceeded to draw a monster/crocodile. He couldn't say much about it, so I asked if it was a funny, nice or bad one. He replied, 'It's everything altogether!' When I wondered where this crocodile came from, he scrutinized me closely. I suggested aloud that it might come from my country. He looked at me intensely out of the corner of his eye and after some hesitation he finally burst out, 'No!' with a shy laugh. I shared his laugh, mine being caring and secure.

His initial transference was a suspicious, questioning one: would I be benevolent (nice), would I accept him enough to smile, or would I devour him, as signified by the spines, teeth and blood that covered the monster/crocodile's mouth and body? Kim himself was like a wild animal on his guard, the prey of persecuting internal objects that he had projected onto me, but the danger he saw in me also had something to do with the realistic danger of his external objects, specifically in the light of the sexual abuse. Notwithstanding the frailty of his defences, however, he had been able to express his fears via a drawing, and I hoped to consolidate this into what Winnicott (1971: 54) once called 'the overlap of the two play areas, that of the patient and that of the therapist'.

This feeling of being under the threat of malevolent internal and external objects, unable to anticipate or master them, soon dominated the transference–countertransference scene. The absence or frailty of appropriate defences, such as repression and displacement, gave a special flavour to our relationship. I felt I could reach so easily to the deepest level of his near-psychotic fears and this was part of the immediate attraction I had in working with him. I also knew that his analysis would involve the same intensity and complexity of feelings for me. But I also knew I would painfully have to receive, accept and hold his projections before working them through for him, so that eventually he could do the same for himself.

For the first six to eight months Kim could not take in interpretations. He was as yet unable to work with the 'as-if' nature of the transference and countertransference. His ego was not structured enough, his thinking was too concrete. My words, to start with, were not experienced as symbols for a fantasy. For example, in our first meeting I could not have referred to his fear of crocodile-me as he would have thought I was about to attack him. In the same way, during our third session, which followed Hallowe'en celebration, he asked what I had been disguised as – 'Maybe a witch?' He looked fearful and I clearly felt he could not differentiate at that moment between me and a witch. This pointed also to his frail sense of reality, the affective power of his fantasies quickly sweeping aside any distinction between reality and fantasy. When I asked what disguise he had worn, he said, 'A zombie!' and he made some grimacing faces. Our 'disguises' were glued to our skins.

Interestingly, the same dynamic between Kim and his objects was paralleled in Kim's mind between words and what they signified. I was struck by the absence of safe distancing between Kim and his objects, the absence of a sense of individuality. In the same manner, there was no clear demarcation between a word and what it signified, no true symbolization. No transitional space was available and I had to be extremely cautious about what I would say and how. Thus, after about a month of therapy, we were playing a game where I was throwing some Lego pieces into a plastic bag held by Kim. He 'ate' them with chewing noises. The game evolved, alongside Kim's excitement but still within bearable limits, into us throwing Lego pieces, aiming at one another's knees. I commented on how important it was to reach each other in this game, and how enjoyable this was for him. I could feel the sexual quality of his excitement and I added that it was as if we were touching one another through this game.

This was too much for Kim, and the game soon became messy, as he started banging all the Lego pieces on the floor. I could sense I had gone too far in addressing the sexual nature of the transference, and that this was equivalent for Kim to acting it out. I realized I could only partially address the transference, keeping in mind its most charged aspects until Kim would be able to verbalize his fantasies. As Rosenfeld and Sprince (1965: 505) commented, when writing about borderline children,

> It therefore soon became clear that our technique had to be modified to facilitate repression and displacement, rather than to make unconscious material conscious. . . . To some extent, because of the nature of the borderline disturbance, our function as therapists must be different and has something of the quality of an auxiliary ego, at least in the initial phase.

Indeed, our first sessions were filled with Kim's sudden outbursts of anxiety. The rapidity with which a game would 'tip over' from pleasure to uncontained anxiety was as confusing to me as it must have been to him. Kim didn't seem able to put much thinking into our games. Whether we were banging cars, jumping or he was trying to lash at my legs with a towel, he kept to this activity until it reached a peak of excitement which then could not be contained. I had agreed to engage with him and share his games within certain clearly defined limits. When it was necessary to step out of these games, particularly when they became organized battles between us, I would put into words what he still could do and what was not reasonable, as in, 'I won't play this game. I won't actually let you hurt me, but instead you can say what it is you want.' He soon made some attempts to verbalize his rage.

However, these boundaries were often difficult for him to maintain and he would quickly become anxiously destructive. He would then lash out, shout at me and tell me I was 'fucking mad', smash all his toys against the wall and aim pens or his fists at me. Sometimes his only way not to 'destroy' me was to leave the room. I felt very much like a fragile dinghy, swept over by a hurricane's waves, desperately needing some anchorage to resist the tempest. One could wonder why I joined in these games, as they almost inevitably led to gross acting-out. To me, playing together was a way of being with Kim on a non-verbal level, trying to protect the pleasure we could share in these games. It was a very primary way of letting him feel that I accepted him. But there was another dimension to these games which I was to discover in time.

Observing Kim's reunions with his mother at the end of our sessions was very revealing to me. Kim would launch himself into mother's arms, have long, loving hugs with her, look intensely into her eyes, as if lost in them. This reminded me of a scene of two lovers meeting up but it was also reminiscent of a reunion between mother and baby. As a matter of fact, Kim would sometimes complain of having 'nappy rash', or try to suck at his mother's breast. She would often be excited by this, press him against her body even tighter, indulging their wish for over-closeness.

The lack of limits in Kim's access to his mother's body had an obvious sexual component. I wondered how much this fuelled a fantasy of merging together. The absence of differentiation not only of their two bodies but also of their two minds prevailed. These exhibitionist displays in the waiting-room, with their exclusive sharing of a common fantasy world, left me excluded. As the third person, possibly the Oedipal rival or simply the living personification of a symbolic differentiation between them, I was left defeated and helpless. In the light of this, it is hardly surprising that Kim often spent his sessions shaking, as if terrified. Being together in the room led to an exciting but deadly fantasy of our merging together, as in the car-banging game. Kim would give me a car, take another sturdier one for himself and we would 'have a go'. He would not elaborate on this game, but would frantically ask for it – 'The game, you know!' The repetitive smashing of the vehicles against one another had a specific value to him, as an exciting collusion between two people, but also as a recapitulation of the abuse in an effort actively to master the trauma. Also, battling with me emptied his mind through its repetitive action at the same time as it gave him some 'saving' distancing from me.

Thus, one day, I suggested a variation to his game: our cars would go under a chair-bridge, then two chair-bridges. Skill and control were required, no banging gratification or ensuing panic. He enjoyed this but he suddenly interrupted the game to sit on my lap. 'Tired,' he said. He rested only a second, before returning to his unrestrained car-banging. I suggested we draw instead, and I drew a head, which he turned into a 'monster-bat'. Then I drew another head, more human, which he rejected angrily. I said perhaps he found this one too much like a boy's head. He began to throw pens and Lego pieces, not at me but at the ceiling.

Even wild animals need a place to rest from time to time, but they have to feel safe to do so. Kim's resting on my lap was very brief before he launched back into his crashing activity. He gave in momentarily and probably absent-mindedly to a need to be close, but the tinge of security was soon swept over by fantasies of being overwhelmed, probably linked with the excitement of sitting on my lap. I felt robbed of a precious moment of caring, and abruptly pushed back into his world of destruction. Throughout his therapy, especially at the beginning, I had to navigate between hope and despair, as Kim's mind oscillated between benevolent and deadly internal objects.

At this early stage in his therapy (the first two months), it became clear that my primary role would be twofold – first, to hold as long as I could on to the content of his fantasies and anxieties before mirroring them back to him, and second, to promote the development of ego functions to help him develop his own capacities by which he would calm his anxieties. In the counter-transference I could experience Kim's relief, his growing trust in me, which lessened his recourse to projections and acting-out.

Working within the triangle of mother, Kim and me

After two months Kim refused to come to his room and for the next two months this shaped our therapeutic sessions; mother, Kim and I began meeting in the waiting-room. There I could observe the way mother overindulged his fantasies. They would get lost in the mutual excitement of this shared togetherness. They would actively exclude me, whispering to each other, Kim lying on his mother, half baby, half sexual partner. I was, in such instances, painfully impotent. Still, there were times when I was the parent, in between them, through my contrasting calmness and attunement with Kim's anxieties.

One of the first occasions when I could sense his inclusion of me and of my role came during an account he gave of a 'nightmare' from the night before; a man, like a robot, had walked towards him, his hand covering Kim's face. Mum exclaimed with enthusiasm, 'Oh! It's like in *Alien!*' Kim was standing between us and he replied, 'Yes! Still, it was a bit scary!' I was moved by the way he tried to verbalize his feelings, and to ward off any deadly engulfment.

We started to have games in the waiting-room where his mother would be the 'ruler'. He drew a 'control machine' for his mother to help him restrain his and her moods. Mother was surprised by these games; she accepted them and reflected on them with a growing understanding of their value. It wasn't long before I saw her anticipate the rapid switch from his exciting embraces of her to his 'killing' attack upon her; she then pointed to a pillow and made it clear he should direct his aggression at this pretend mother, and not any more at her. I became convinced that this strange triangle had been a saving one, not only for Kim, but for his mother and for the therapy. Kim had included her in the work, and she had used it to reflect on his being a separate individual, and to accept my role more. The mutually alienating dynamic between them had started to shift.

With hindsight, I think that the basis of our work in the first six to eight months of therapy had evolved around his perception of my holding capacity and his acceptance and use of new psychic tools. I could integrate his projections, without 'comfortably' turning them back to him, waiting until he would be ready to explore them more with me.

One day, Kim had started the session by crawling up the stairs to my room, making 'barmy' faces, in quite a provocative way. Once in the room, he took some pieces of balsa-wood from his box and threw them in my direction, trying to scare me, which I verbalized. To this, he asked if he had scared me. I commented on how important it was to him to be able to do so. He then made up a 'game' in which we would fight each other. I tried to 'open up' the game up by asking questions like what names we should have, where we came from, etc. He was much stronger than me and I commented on how nice it must feel to be strong, able to defend oneself, instead of being weak and frightened. This was the only way Kim could listen to me. I chose not to talk of his own fear of being 'barmy', as he would call it, but of how uneasy it was to feel vulnerable, in danger, unable to protect oneself, like me in the game. My attempts at 'opening' the game up were aimed at using it in our work, as a displaced representation of the transference. It is noteworthy that his physical and mental tension lowered as he was more able to work in displacement. I could use what I felt in the countertransference, but without reflecting it back to him as his feelings. I knew that this step would have to be taken, but later. The countertransference was a suffering one. I felt as if I had to hold the quivering pieces of a jigsaw together, give it a more solid basis. I offered him a model of my mind, which he needed to internalize before any interpretative work could start.

In one of his early sessions, Kim sang, in a reverie, 'No one understands my mind!' After six months, he had the following joke:

'What's your name?'
'Beatrice.'
'What's this?' – pointing to his nose.
'Nose.'
'What's in my hands?' – opening them.
'Nothing.'
'Exactly! Beatrice knows nothing!'

I smiled. Our treatment alliance was established! There was a sense of him letting me know his trust in my care, as if he started to trust his own potentially good, internal world. He was now also able to sublimate his omnipotence and aggression in ways more appropriate to his age.

Development of Kim's ego and the 'thinking therapist' game

After about six months Kim's mother reported some improvement in her son. He was more 'sure of himself', 'had been able to walk on a trunk, over a river, without any help'. He was quieter at home, could tolerate frustration better and would spend hours building balsa-wood models. His behaviour at school was still problematic: he was still the 'barmy', 'handicapped' one, actively rejected by others. Mother was intrigued by this discrepancy, and was inclined to attribute it to the school's lack of understanding of her son rather than to his difficulties.

In the sessions, my overall feeling was of a quieter child; the 'boat' was more stable, its hull less permeable to his internal tempests, as if the latter had lessened in intensity. As he was more able to hold his mind together, I spent less of my time holding him in mine. From about eight to ten months of therapy, as his ego developed in strength and structure, he was more accepting of us as two separate individuals with two separate bodies and minds, and he could start working at the symbolic level of inter-pretations. This change was fascinating to observe.

The sessions were still governed by his chaotic swings of mood and his prevalent use of projections. Still, a slight thread of conti-nuity began to develop between bits of sessions which I tried to encourage as much as I could. This was centred on using my own countertransference to tell him what I was thinking and feeling, without interpreting his projections directly, so that he could observe it and explore it within the safety of not having to own it quite yet. I tried to use his projections as a basis of reflecting aloud on 'myself', e.g. 'How come I am so "barmy" [his word] today? It is so upsetting to feel confused, not to be able to control one's feelings.' I was held by the silent complicity of his smile or, even better, by his attentive listening. I was giving him the opportunity to follow, and hopefully internalize my own efforts at understanding bits of 'myself', thinking them over for him.

This thread of verbalizing my thoughts was also followed in guessing games introduced by Kim. The prevalence of magical thinking in Kim was such that he was usually very anxious about my guessing what was in his mind, but as with his need to test out the issue of closeness, so he constantly initiated these games as a test. I would have to guess what number he was thinking of, and if I got it wrong his triumph was commensurate only with his terror if I got it right. He would then withdraw implacably. These guessing games prevailed at the time when he was about to come back to the consulting-room. I had to take part in them, knowing that his margin of safety was extremely thin and vulnerable.

Little by little, I tried to give some flexibility to those games, commenting on the fallibility of my mind, e.g. 'Oh! Silly me! I did not guess the right number! If only my mind was magic I would have got it right!' Another game consisted of him covering his drawings with his left hand; I had to guess what they were.

He would lift up his 'shield' only for a fraction of a second and ask me defiantly what he had just drawn. Most of the time I could not guess correctly and I would comment, to his satisfaction, on my own limits. I would also on occasion express my own frustration playfully, but also genuine thoughtfulness, which Kim listened to with amusement and attention. He would enjoy such comments as, 'Oh! I did not guess! How frustrating! I would feel so good if I could win all the time, but I can't!' I would play it up a bit, making my own states of mind more perceptible to him. These simple games did not, of course, totally reduce his recourse to magical thinking. At best, I hoped to ease some confusion over my mental power. Most of all, it gave me a very nice opportunity to work on such themes as magical thinking, ego limits, labelling of feelings, reality and wishes differentiation. Addressing his anxiety directly would only have confirmed for him the overwhelming power of my mind, so that I had to find lighter, more 'playful' methods which gave him a choice about taking in the essence of my words or not. In any case, through the playfulness of my comments, I tacitly offered a respectful space between my words and what he would hear. This gave him the chance to start thinking apart himself, without me fully 'knowing'.

Towards object-constancy, separation – individuation and symbolic representation

It was noticeable that at about the same stage in his therapy (eight to ten months), Kim made up other games, in which he would gauge the closeness between us.

For example, as he separated from his mother in the waiting-room, he would run upstairs towards the consulting-room, and I was to follow him, not too close, but not too far away either. There was a lot of excitement in this. From what I could feel of his emotional state, coupled with my own associations, this game had a tremendous importance. Being chased was highly exciting to him, but not without a fearful component. If I was too close to him, near enough to 'catch him', he would shout at me to stop, to 'fuck off'. A variation of this game consisted of me walking behind him up the stairs, adopting the stamping rhythm of his feet on the steps. I was 'crap' if I couldn't do it exactly, but if my rhythm corresponded too closely to his, he would get into a panic-rage. 'We're different, we're not the same!' he would retort.

It seemed to me that too much proximity, either mental as in the guessing game, or physical as in the racing game, or more symbolic perhaps as in the last game, would entail an incommensurate anxiety for Kim. My own associations with these enactments of Kim's fantasies evolved around his fear of being invaded by me, or attacked in a devouring way. However, it seemed that these games had a creative value as well in bringing a useful field of experimentations to our meetings. With these games, Kim could discover, at his own pace, what the separation between two individuals meant – having two separate minds, two separate bodies, playing with this difference as a possibility for him to exist in himself without being overwhelmed by death anxieties. I took an active position in these games, playing up his enjoyment and surprise at being two separate individuals sharing the 'simple' pleasure of a game. Through these games Kim began actively to master the possibility of attempting to regulate the distance between himself and the other.

Kim began to internalize a constant object, which permitted him in turn to sustain his growing sense of a separate individuality. To his regression and distress at any coming break, I would acknowledge his feeling of loss, but also I would build for him a sense of my holding him in mind with interest, beyond the threat of interruptions. Loss became less acute with time, as he could hold on to a consistent image of me, and of himself too.

The best illustration of this came after a year of treatment. He had started building a balsa-wood boat just before the summer break. I talked about the pain we would both feel at not seeing each other for six weeks. He was very regressed and paranoid at this time and he used the boat construction as a way of isolating himself from me, which I respected. He added bits to this mysterious boat every day, sometimes throwing it at the walls in a desperate rage, blaming me for its destruction. He still managed, however, to hang on to it until his last day, letting me put it in his locker, where 'it would be safe'. At that stage, he called the construction a 'security gun'. I did not speak of it as a defence against loss, but as a precious asset when one feels in danger.

To my surprise, on his first day back, he took the construction out and converted it slowly into a boat, a 'Chinese junk', as he called it. He was calmer, as if holding more benevolent objects inside himself, ones that would not get lost over time but would stay safely enough inside him. He worked on this boat for several weeks, until one day he smashed it against the wall. I think he had perceived my too strong attachment to it. My pleasure in his forward move had frightened him, as if he had seen in it some threat, possibly the 'loving' engulfment by his primal object. By breaking the boat, he had pulled me back, abruptly, to his darker side. I had been too quick for him, confusing an intimate hope for him to get better with a given fact, and he had punished me for this *faux pas*.

Since then, covering the second year of treatment, there had been an evolving theme in his sessions: from the broken junk, Kim spent many weeks engrossed in wasps, then in birds' bones, paper planes and finally seeds. This long journey, from destructive internal objects to creativity and birth, went along with the strengthening of his ego and his internalization of a constant and benevolent object. After 18 months of intensive therapy, Kim's ego depended less on my auxiliary ego.

One of the first sessions after the long summer break, about a year within therapy, Kim wanted us to play chess, copying each other. The game soon became confusing. He tried to trick me in order to win, and threw his king down with false rage. He emptied out the contents of his box of toys with deliberate provocation. I commented on how in the past he used to lose his control so often, whereas now he could choose and let me know of this new ability. He smiled and picked up his balsa-wood boat, the Chinese junk he had started before the break. He asked me to glue some boards on the side. He said he had started it 'a year ago' and I commented on his patience, and also on how this boat had waited for him during the holidays.

This short sequence provides a sense of Kim's growing control over his drives and his own acknowledgement of inner feelings. It also shows the development of object-constancy (his pride at having started the boat a year earlier), and his trust in me. His use of magical thinking gradually reduced. He was able to some degree to contain his anxiety, defend against it, and express his feelings in a more verbalized way. Going along with John Steiner's (1979) thoughts on the interrelationship between letting go of the concrete object in the process of mourning and the ability to set up a symbolic representation, one could suggest that Kim's new psychological assets enabled him to reach a different level of functioning, where it was possible to analyse his conflicts and his use of defences.

With his access to symbolic representations, my work was much easier. I could start interpreting the material without dreading too much his anxious regressed response. Within the triangle of Kim, his mother and me, we had been able to facilitate the process for his internal growth. This led to the exciting possibility of working 'analytically' on his conflicts, defences, fantasies within a safe enough transferential–countertransferential relationship.

After a year of 'preparation', he expressed directly his anxiety that I would attack the wasps, which he liked, and kill them. I would also destroy his paper planes if I touched them. Little by little he could verbalize his fears and he opened up to my words as well. In displacement first, then directly, he could voice his fear that I would 'sex' him: 'You'll eat my penis, you'll destroy it!' There were echoes of his first session but in a different form. He voiced the mixture of excitement and anxiety about our being together in the room as 'the banging car game can be dangerous!' and then he gave that game up altogether. He seemed slowly to relinquish the transference re-enactment of the experience of abuse.

At the end of one session, during the time he said I would 'sex' him, he exhibited his locker key, held as a penis, to his mother in the waiting-room. I took this up the next day as we were starting to build up some planes, commenting on the significance of the key as a penis, and noticing how much we had talked about this issue recently. He asked if I had ever had sex. I related this to his curiosity and possible concern about sexual matters. I linked it with what had happened when, as a child, he was sexually attacked by a 'friend'. He asked me if I was handicapped. I took up his fear that I would do the same to him as this boy had done. He seemed a bit more relaxed and went on with his plane, calling it a 'spotted hyena', showing me a drawing he had made on the wing (a squiggle). He wanted to make another plane called 'the serpent' and this created a bit of a distance between us, but it had also been permitted by his lessened tension as we talked about his fears within the transference. His exhibitionism with his mother from the day before did not return. The general feeling was that words had been able to contain him, to give him an instrument to stop his acting-out, to have recourse to other ways of being, and mainly to do some working through of his anxieties.

While there was less acting-out and while Kim could, with my help, express more of his feelings, there was still a balance to keep, or the boat would tip over. The feeling I had was of a growth

towards separation–individuation. With his mother's encouragement he started making friends at school and he was invited
overnight and enjoyed it, managing the separation from mother.
His schoolwork improved, though he was still receiving special
needs help. At the age of 10, although slightly anxious, he was
proud to announce that he could take the bus to and from school
by himself. These events were confirmation of internal changes.

Some recent material: further separation and managing his exclusion from my mother/baby dyad

As a starting point for more thinking about this child, I would like
to give some extracts of very recent material, as Kim is now
confronted with my pregnancy which, as one might imagine,
would be an extremely charged issue for him.

I had chosen to tell him I was going to have a baby when I
was five months pregnant, as a way to frame his expected anxiety,
and also as I knew that his fantasies would need a long time to
unravel and be worked through. I initially felt some relief in him,
as if the presence of a 'third' between us could dilute his regressive pull to merge with me. There was also some expression of
concern – 'You can't run any more' – but signs of distress came
steadily, starting with very discreet ones, such as his wondering
if the piece of balsa-wood he was manipulating would break, to
wild enactment. I would like to present some material from the
second session following my disclosure.

As I picked him up from the waiting-room, he greeted me by
pointing to his stomach, asking by gestures if I had told his mother
yet. He spent some time in the toilet and came out, his hair well
brushed, looking quite boyish. Once in the room, he ate an elongated ice-cream. He sat opposite me on the couch, and we played
a made-up game, using the chess board and pieces. It was a
complicated battle-like game, in which our pieces had specific
moves, the pieces being closely grouped together to start with.
There was something withdrawn in his concentration on the game,
as well as a clear wish to defeat me which made me feel helpless. We had both been given a 'magic pawn'. He quickly got
hold of mine, asking me how I could lose it. I asked what he
would do if he had a 'magic pawn' in his life. He bounced a chess
piece in his hand anxiously.

After a pause, I suggested he might find it difficult to be with me today, because of what we had spoken about two days earlier. He talked over me, wiped some chess pieces and went to the sink where he spat. He then went to his locker to fetch his 'tar baby' (a doll he had covered in black paint). He called me a 'witch' and bashed the baby on the table and armchairs. He became excited and showed me the doll's face, exclaiming that the bumps had not left a mark. He seemed fascinated, repeating this activity again. I intervened to say that his wish to hurt my baby, even if he had such an idea, would not hurt for real. This was a way of reassuring him in his struggle to express his aggressive feelings. 'I know!' he replied and later he added, 'I don't want to!' yet he went on bashing the doll up with rage.

After a while I said that some children in his position might feel let down; they would think of me as a 'witch' and would like to get rid of the baby. I added that I could understand such feelings. I put it like this because I felt I had given him the 'permission' to be aggressive, and now I had to help him put these strong feelings into words. He continued bashing the baby until the end of the session. When the session ended he stopped and left, without answering to my 'goodbye'.

It seems that Kim will be able to overcome the pain involved in my pregnancy and unusually long absence. Many feelings and fantasies have come up – the intensity of his rage, his sense of loss, his jealousy of the baby, his wish to replace the father. These fantasies might galvanize his therapy if I am able to contain his anxiety and moderate the pace and rhythm of the work at the same time as addressing and working through his distress.

Conclusion

I have described some of the technical issues involved in working with a child with severe ego impairment. When such a child is overwhelmed by fantasies, his fragile ego is unable to sustain them, so that he easily regresses to psychotic-like states of mind. When his object relatedness lacks constancy, swinging from rejection to merging, then the child is deprived of what Fred Pine (1974: 348) calls 'The basic stabilisers of functioning that other children acquire: a reliable anchor in external reality and in patterned object-relationships that give them shape, and an array of intra-psychic defences reliably set into motion when anxiety is aroused'. One of my first aims was to enable Kim to develop such 'stabilisers' which could assist him and then facilitate interpretative work.

The very steady input of intensive treatment has allowed him to use me as a containing, constant and structuring external object, something he had previously lacked. It has also enabled his mother to become containing, thus stabilizing more of his external world. Kim has, to some extent, become able to modify and manage his own wild fluctuations of internal states, to take over some of my functions. Stemming from this, he has been able to release and work on the 'killing' power of his internal objects, projected on to me or others.

After two years Kim has come a long way but he is still far from being able to contain his feelings enough and to verbalize them instead of acting them out. We have not yet tamed his internal 'crocodile-monster'. The echoes of his wild internal states still preoccupy his mind, and my own, which suggests that the days of the 'Chinese junk', graceful and serene, may yet need a long time to sail into view.

Acknowledgement

I wish to acknowledge the contributions made by Audrey Gavshon and Viviane Green to the writing of this chapter.

Chapter 7

Caught inside a web

Some technical formulations around working at the 'psychotic' border

Lesley Pover

Introduction

This chapter reports on some of the technical issues that were thrown up in the psychotherapy of an 8-year-old girl, whom I shall call Gemma, with severe ego impairment. Gemma was a troubled child who suffered a series of shocking experiences early in life which left her with a legacy of disturbance – self-injurious behaviour, emotional storms, violence, chanting, head-bobbing, and fluctuations between states of terror and excited hyperarousal. During her sessions Gemma was also prone to being drawn towards objects in the therapy room that released her from her grip on reality. As her therapist I found these moments shocking, but they were also experienced by me as moments in which the highly compressed contents of her traumas were being unpacked. Therapeutically I was then required to perform, as a mother with a normal infant would, certain ego functions and ego-supporting functions on her behalf. In addition, certain *reality-finding* functions had to be performed to combat the child's perverse reliance on some of the secondary gains of her psychotic moments. This involved the technique of active injunctions to the child in a way that has been similarly employed in work with some autistic children (Tustin 1981; Alvarez 1992) and with some borderline adult patients with massive developmental arrest (Little 1981; Gedo and Gehrie 1993).

By those who knew her best Gemma was considered an enigmatic child. Her capacity for attachment was intense, the feelings evoked and projected ranging from genuine compassion to hostility. Gemma's sudden and unpredictable outbursts of violence towards herself or others and her inconsolable states of terror, which also tended to end in outbursts of violence or ritualistic chanting, made caring for her difficult. As she grew, so did her capacity to damage herself and those around her. The desire to refer her for psychotherapy was strong and those responsible were tenacious in their efforts. I believe this was partly born out of the desperation of not understanding or knowing how to help her but also out of a hopeful feeling that she could be helped.

Panting followed by head-bobbing have always been the signals that Gemma was unhappy. Her movements were rhythmic, and at the climax there was an explosion of uncontrollable behaviour that included head-banging. When she became unsure and anxious she masturbated for reassurance but this often led to disturbing states of excitement. Along with this behaviour Gemma frequently became aggressively excited when she saw others in distress. To be alone with Gemma was also considered risky. A lot of work was therefore undertaken to ensure that those involved in caring for Gemma – her mother and step-father, Social Services and the Child Protection Team – understood the therapeutic process, which at some stage would involve negative feelings towards me. Before I met Gemma for an assessment I waded through the mountain of documentation on her life and also met some of the adults who knew her best. All this information was helpful but it did not prepare me for our first meeting or for the relationship that developed. One person mentioned that Gemma was a pretty child and liked to be admired, a small piece of descriptive information that I forgot until we met.

Family history

Gemma was born hypotonic but her mother felt a strong bond with this floppy, helpless infant, possibly because she too saw herself as defenceless and vulnerable, trapped in an unhappy, extremely volatile marriage. For the first two and a half years, until Gemma learnt to walk, she was carried around in her mother's arms. Mother talked with great affection about this period. The bonding was strong, she said, the two were quite inseparable. However, this meant that Gemma, as a babe in arms, was a witness to, and no doubt felt a part of, a great deal of domestic violence.

Early medical reports mention that in the first few months of life Gemma reached some normal milestones (not specified). It was not until she was 7 months old that concerns were raised about developmental delays. Initially it was thought that extra stimulation was needed, but by 15 months more serious behaviour had developed. Gemma had changed from a placid, floppy baby to one who shrieked at eye contact. She had begun to pull her hair out and scratch her skin till it bled, and she started headbanging. For a time Gemma had arm splints and for a number of years wore a leather helmet.

At 2½ she was assessed and at that time a diagnosis of Rett's syndrome with some 'autistic' features was made (later discounted). Investigations into epilepsy confirmed that she did experience some epileptic activity. As a result Gemma was placed on medication; the last recorded seizure was noted when she was 4 years old. EEGs since have shown no signs of epilepsy.

The arrival of a new baby in the family soon after Gemma's third birthday was a terrible shock for her. Mother described the look of horror on her daughter's face; it was something she would never forget. Gemma needed constant attention and this role was being increasingly carried out by daily helpers. Social Services also offered support by periodically arranging temporary foster care in order to give other family members a rest. Shortly after her fourth birthday, while in foster care, Gemma managed to run out of the house and, although she did not go far, she became lost. She was running across a busy road when she was hit by a double-decker bus. From material constructed in therapy it is likely that she witnessed this large vehicle bearing down upon her. It took some time to extricate her from under the bus but apparently she did not lose consciousness until she was in the ambulance. She suffered severe lacerations and several broken bones, but no head injuries.

The result of the accident initially had a calming effect upon her. There was less head-banging and generally she was quieter. Mother felt that for many months she was in a state of shock. Whilst there was a reduction in the amount of self-mutilation, the attacks on her sibling increased.

The situation became more serious as Gemma grew older and the family's circumstances changed. Mother went through an acrimonious divorce and shortly after remarried. Within a couple of years there were two more babies. The ferocity of Gemma's headbanging returned but those who were getting hurt now included the adults who cared for her. They could be injured while trying to protect Gemma during an outburst or when intervening to prevent her from attacking a sibling.

An assessment was again undertaken when Gemma was 6 years old and this confirmed the lack of integration in her development that had been noted before. Some 'autistic features' were still apparent (the need for sameness of routines and a number of bizarre rituals) but she demonstrated more advanced levels of imaginative play and social interaction than an autistic child. Her IQ score was 50 and language and comprehension were found to be severely delayed – her non-verbal score was 3 years, and her capacity to use words symbolically was also limited. For example, some phrases such as 'cut it out', meaning stop or withdraw, would be experienced as a potential attack. She feared that 'it' literally had to be physically cut out of her. Other words had strong associations. The word 'appointment', for example, would cause her to scream because this meant a visit to the doctor or dentist, which for Gemma were terrifying places. Once when I used the word 'prepare' she ran and crouched in a corner. From this position she told me she did not like the word 'pair/pear' as it got under her skin. Gemma has always attended special educational schools but the view of her abilities has changed since the commencement of psychotherapy. She is seen as more capable and skilled than tests would suggest. The view presently held is that her capacity to learn is impeded by emotional rather than intellectual factors. Her current problems fit a diagnosis of 'mixed psychopathology' (Towbin *et al.* 1993), leaning towards what Pine (1974) has termed the 'psychotic border' of children with borderline disturbance.

The assessment period

During my three assessment meetings with Gemma I was to gain a clearer impression of her ego impairments and some of the extreme anxieties which assailed her sense of self. For the first session she was accompanied by her mother. When I went to meet her she was sitting quietly next to her mother in the waiting-room. Despite the mass of curly blonde hair I was shocked by her appearance – the hard red callus at the back of her skull (created through years of head-banging which had distorted the shape of her head), her downcast eyes and the twisted features of her face. It was not the child I expected to see. The remark about her attractiveness, made by one of the helpers, came back to me and I wondered how anyone could think of this child as pretty.

Although only a momentary reaction, the visual impact on me was one of shock, instinctive withdrawal and a feeling of repulsion. Gemma's downcast eyes and her faltering gait, like that of a disabled child, were possibly what she wanted me to see or even expected me to see. (In reality she was quite an attractive child, agile and at times extremely dextrous.) I felt that she knew all too well my inward reaction.

Sinason (1992) has described how a primary handicap can be compounded by the reactions and primitive emotional contact of the infant/mother dyad. If the mother unconsciously conveys her feelings of shock, withdrawal, disappointment, and a legion of other feelings, what does the infant make of his/her first meeting and what is internalized? If thoughts about the damaged child cannot be processed, which includes mourning the loss of the healthy child, then Sinason suggests there is a danger of a secondary handicap developing.

Our journey from the waiting-room to the therapy room was a slow and difficult one, with Gemma making several attempts to run away. As we entered the room she held tightly on to her mother's hand. She took two steps into the room and suddenly stopped. Her gaze was now firmly on me. She stood with her back against the wall and pushed her head forward. There was a short, sharp bobbing movement of the head, then her knees momentarily gave way and her whole body jerked up and down. As she bobbed she asked me if she could leave. I commented on how everything must seem strange and new to her – the room, the toys and me. She uttered a solitary cry: 'No Pover for Gemma! No Pover!' While maintaining the tight grip on her mother, she slid down the wall and with her other hand she began to pull her hair and bang her head against the wall.

I spoke slowly, quietly but firmly and said I could see her distress and how the newness and strangeness terrified her. I explained that I was going to stay where I was and that if I moved I would tell her first. She listened and was momentarily satisfied with my response but I could see she was still anxious and watchful. From her crouched position she looked small, vulnerable and very frightened.

She asked if I was about to become her new carer. She was probably fearful that I was going to take her away and that the clinic would be her new temporary home.

When the feelings of terror subsided she left her mother and began to explore the room. The exploration was of a sensual nature which involved tapping, pulling and feeling the furniture as if to ensure its safety. From the tapping I gained a sense that this was not only about some worry about the solidity of the furniture. I felt she was getting to 'know' the furniture like someone who was visually impaired. Once she relaxed she was able to tell me how frightened she was that the furniture and toys would 'jump out and hurt her'. During this first meeting she also seemed to be testing the physical boundaries designed for her safety by making various attempts to escape from the room and explore the rest of the building.

In the second session Gemma showed me how part of her personality was attracted to frightening and potentially dangerous situations. After one of her many explorations of the room she tried hard to open a large locked cupboard. She told me she had one just like it. She pulled the handle vigorously in an attempt to open it and laughed as she told me that being in the cupboard meant 'getting lost', and that this was fun. From the cupboard she moved to the disused gas fire and began to play with one of the taps. When I disapproved she headed for an electric socket. I thought she wanted to show me that she knew what was dangerous.

Despite her attraction to these dangerous places, I thought she was interested in my response, and it seemed that only after she had experienced my firmness about what was safe and what was not was there any attempt at play. She moved to the large doll's house and managed to pick up a few small dolls from her box. She opened the front door for the mummy doll and said she was going up the stairs. But her attention was drawn to the small front door. She tapped and pushed at the small square Perspex window on the door. She exerted more pressure until the small pane fell out. She was unperturbed and she explained that this 'was for the noise to come in'. I asked 'What noise?' She replied, 'The noise of the traffic'. I asked if she was frightened by it and she nodded. Looking at the house she said 'Hoover' and confirmed that this noise frightened her too. Later in the session she mentioned that the noise from outside didn't always frighten her, sometimes she was 'all right'. Her interest, though, had shifted from the small door to the square of Perspex. She tasted it and tried to break off a corner of it. I had seen enough.

I reflected the events and stated how I was going to intervene to stop further damage from taking place. She snapped 'No!' and tried to replace the Perspex. I watched while she made vain attempts to replace it in the door. She became exhausted and without a word she limply handed me the pane. I felt that she was showing me her fragility, how she had very little protection from being bombarded from external and internal stimuli. For her there was no way of totally shutting them out or keeping them in. Nevertheless, she seemed to have an awareness that some things came from outside while other events were internal disturbances. In the above play I was reminded of Freud's concept of the contact-barrier, later developed by Bion (1962a). If the Perspex is taken as representing the permeable contact-barrier between conscious and unconscious, and if this is then damaged, there is little resistance to the passage of elements from one zone to the other. Frequently I noticed how an unexpected noise made Gemma jump, as if she experienced the sound as getting right inside her. On other occasions when she was about to have an outburst she would say she 'wanted to stay Gemma'.

Throughout the assessment period I was aware of Gemma's acute interest in me – in what I was going to allow in the room and in my emotional state. In addition, I was beginning to feel that there was an aspect of her personality committed to worrying and disturbing people. I was also struck by the intensity and suddenness of emotional changes. These changes were constant and often very subtle. The more obvious swings were from states of terror to a sudden perverse enjoyment of placing herself in danger. The often subtle moment-to-moment shifts in intense emotions were conflict-free; previous states appeared to be instantly forgotten. In developmental terms I was reminded of a much younger child who has little capacity for self-reflectiveness. The same could be said for her method of exploration, which was essentially of a tactile nature, normally associated with the infantile stage.

Beginning of treatment

Gemma was seen in three times per week therapy, and, because of her acute states of terror during the assessment period, I had envisaged that it would take time before she was prepared to be alone with me. But this was not the case. The impetus for change came from her during the first week of her therapy when she required the presence of her escort in the room for brief moments only. What became more important was the knowledge that they were there and waiting for her. At first they waited in the corridor outside the therapy room but within a few months she was happy for them to stay in the waiting-room.

Gemma, however, remained fragile. Her states of mind fluctuated rapidly. Generally it was imperative for me to hold on to her feelings and not reflect them back too quickly. The importance of language and how and when to communicate, and at what level, was as much a matter of intuition as technique. If I got it wrong, and at times I did, it would whip her up into a state where she could easily physically attack me or an object within the room. For example, if I said something like 'You want to hurt me because you're feeling hurt', she would hear it as a confirmation, giving her permission to proceed. I think she was also telling me I had not got the message – she *needed* me to feel the hurt. Yet for her to experience being understood often implied more than getting the words right. At times of high arousal it was particularly noticeable how she used all her senses. She scanned her surroundings or simply stared at objects; she seemed to feel and smell the atmosphere in a sensual way. Intuitively I used simple phrases like 'Calm down, just calm down', and these worked best when said rhythmically, the pitch of my voice matching the highs and lows of her breathing rate. It worked best of all if I was calm and unruffled and could start speaking at the rhythm of her breathing rate, and take her down slowly. To emphasize the message I would raise and lower my hands so that these too were in unison with my voice. Schore (1996), in describing how interactions with the caregiver help to modulate heightened levels of arousal in the baby, referred to this process as 'down-regulating', and many sessions were spent simply getting her into a less agitated state.

There was, however, another side to Gemma, which never failed to impress me. This was her sense of expectation. Something within her had not given up hope of being understood. Whenever she took my hand to walk to the therapy room her grip was firm and this was indicative of the quality of our relationship. She expected me to be totally involved, constantly attentive, and at times when I followed the rhythm of her breathing, imperceptibly connected to herself. During the early days she would use me as a physical extension of herself, telling me exactly what I should do. The adhesive quality of our relationship reminded me of Gemma's early relationship with her mother, when the two of them were inseparable. However, while it was important for her to be physically close to me, this often resulted in antagonism towards me. I realized that when she was up close she could only see parts of me – my nose, eyes or just my hair; I had become a part-object. I would then gently point out that she was too near and could lose sight of the whole of me, and therefore needed to step back. Timing was all-important in this type of intervention but it always prevented a merger and brought about a me–not me differentiation without the need for violence.

Following other periods of intense interaction I could often sense her drifting away. There were different qualities to this drifting away. Sometimes I had the feeling that, like a small child, she was just exhausted and needed a break to recover. At other times I felt she withdrew because an experience had become too intense. But the link that triggered these distinct responses frequently eluded me. Then on other occasions when she drifted or 'slipped' away I felt she was falling into an abyss of nothingness, and this could have a strangely perverse quality. During these moments she would turn away and gently tap the surface next to her. I found that if I called her name softly, as if waking a small child, I could retrieve her and she would respond by turning and smiling at me.

I wish to describe one occasion, which was to initiate a critical theme in the therapy, where she drifted away but invited me to follow her to the destination she had in mind. She had been tapping mindlessly on the window and she called me over and pointed to the window and said, 'Look, I want to be there.' I looked out of the window and saw the gravel path, the cat lying in the sun, the house next door, the tree next to the window, the busy street below, all of which were within her view. 'No, no,' she said patiently and tugged at my sleeve. 'Look here.' I crouched down beside her and adjusted my vision. There, on the other side of the window-pane, almost indiscernible in the sunlight, was a spider's web. 'The spider's web?' I asked. 'There, there,' she repeated more urgently. I looked and saw she was referring to one of the holes in the web. It seemed to be an entrance, her way of entering another world devoid of time, space, or gravity.

I was later to learn that spiders and spiders' webs had a special meaning for her. I found the metaphor of the spider's web a useful way of thinking about how Gemma processed her emotional experiences. Many of her early life experiences had remained stuck in the web of her mind – her helmet, blood on her skin, the accident. She had not been able to make any sense of these ex-periences, nor had she been able to forget them. The full impact of these experiences could be triggered by comments or incidents in the room that at the time seemed quite random, and then the past would come very much to life in the present. Once, after an involuntary jerk, she stared at her legs and told me she could see blood. At other times she would suddenly frantically lash out at every object within her reach as if her very existence depended upon it. It was easy to think of such emotional 'reminders' as finding a 'fast track' down the spokes of the web to the very hub, messages sent with such speed and ferocity that they rocked the whole structure. The condensation of time and events meant there was little room for new experiences to exist in their own right. Helping her to gain a perspective about what was happening here and now and distinguishing this from what happened a long time ago became an important focus of the work.

Getting to know the trauma

The following extract from shortly before our first long break is taken from a time when Gemma had been in treatment three months. As soon as I entered the waiting-room I became aware that Gemma was on edge and in a state of hyperarousal. She had no shoes on and her escort was holding a quilt used during outbursts to help protect Gemma from hard surfaces. The escort accompanied us to the therapy room and as usual seated herself outside. Gemma had tapped her way along the corridor. Once the escort was seated, Gemma bobbed her head forward and asked repeatedly for reassurance that 'it' was not for her. The escort confirmed that this was so. Gemma bobbed again and told us that 'it' had happened a long time ago. The escort sighed and said that 'it' was nothing to do with her. Such conversations were not unusual as people frequently experienced difficulty in knowing what Gemma was referring to. However, today I felt Gemma was trying to communicate her thoughts.

I asked her if she could tell us what had happened a long time ago. A fixed sadistic smile crept across her face. She pushed her folded tongue out so that she looked grotesque like a gargoyle and flapped her arms. Her whole body stiffened and in a squeaky voice she said she was once hit by a big bus. She began giggling and said that there was blood on her legs. I responded by firmly telling her that 'it' was now over, 'it' was not funny but was probably frightening. She calmed down, the moment passed, and we continued with the session.

Later she asked me to help her search her box for some toys to play 'pass the parcel'. The box was placed between us and as I glanced down Gemma let out an inhuman screech. Startled, I looked up, and she sprang forward and tore her nails down the front of my jumper. Her cry was a piercing one but the incident was over in seconds. I was shaken and stunned and for a moment unable to speak or move. She looked unruffled and continued as if nothing had happened.

Towards the end of the session she began to cry and said she did not want to leave and in her upset state she mentioned eating a cake that had spiders in it. I wondered whether she was experiencing the break as my abandoning her to an 'it' that would destroy her as I left. The latter part of the session had certainly evoked in me the impact of the double-decker bus. Later I began to think of her inhuman cry as possibly representing the screeching of brakes, and her attempts to scratch my jumper as an enactment of the lacerations she received. But in the session these links to the past eluded me.

Eventually it was Gemma's fascination with the visible scar on her stomach which gave me a clue. I had been thinking that it must have required several stitches when the images of the threads sticking up from her stomach suddenly reminded me of spiders. As a confused and traumatized child, what did she think they were? Did she think that she had taken in something really bad and it was now trying to crawl out?

As therapy progressed Gemma became more consciously aware that I was open and available to understanding her and her world. Two of her sessions routinely fell close together, one late in the afternoon and the next session early the following morning. Frequently during these particular sessions she elected to communicate an important experience. I learnt that the prelude to such an experience often started with the question, 'Are you coming to see me tomorrow?' She was aware that physically she came to see me but I felt the question implied my visiting her world.

The following session will illustrate how Gemma continued to unpack the compressed details of her trauma. She sat on top of the tall filing cabinet with her back towards me. She casually swept aside the leaves of the plant which occupied the space next to her.

For a few seconds she sat with her thumb in her mouth and seemed lost in thought. Slowly she turned round and told me that she was going to smash the china plant pot. In an animated tone she said it would go 'smash!' and would cut her all over. She indicated this by pointing at her head and working her way down her body. 'It would cut me here and here and here,' she said. I gave what sounded like a stereotyped interpretation with a paranoid implication: that she was angry with the pot for being in the room all the time and wanted to break it, but if she did she was concerned that the pot would get its own back and smash her up. She nodded one of her slow, exaggerated, disabled-looking nods – mirroring perhaps the inadequacy of my attempts to grasp her meaning. But then she suddenly jerked back to life and excitedly began to tell me again the story of her accident when she was hit by the bus, only this time a more detailed picture emerged as she described glass breaking.

My own intelligence sprang back into life as the link between the impact, the spider, the hole, and states of terror became apparent to me. I realized that she was describing what happens in slow motion to glass when an object hits it: the cracking which spreads as if alive, the web effect, the hole that appears in the spider's body which grows and into which all the bits fall. Her experience was not simply of glass breaking but of it coming to life and attacking her. The impact of the description hit me as if I too had been sent flying through the air. Even though my interpretation about the china pot had perhaps addressed intellectually the consequences of a massive projection, at an emotional level I began to realize how it was possible for inanimate objects to turn instantaneously into dangerous living things.

After wandering round the room she sat on the desk. Her voice changed and in a high pitch she sang to me about layers of toffee and treacle with icing on top. In a squeaky voice she said a hole had appeared in the mixture. She added that it wasn't very nice. I could make nothing of this communication apart from the fact that it sounded sticky and she was excited. I saw her body tense, however, and she pulled her gargoyle face and slowly began to chew her tongue. She had slipped deep into a sticky world and I felt something masochistic was going on. In horror I said, 'You're down there, aren't you?' She glared coldly at me, opened the drawer next to her, and threw hard pieces of play dough in my direction, which in the previous session she had said were faeces.

She now emerged from her sticky world and she suggested we play schools. I was to play the part of a helpless child. I had dirtied myself but after being cleaned up I was taken to the school hall where I was told to sit. She held my hands and informed me I had been naughty. She talked coherently about my pretty dress and asked why I had wet myself (I was slightly dirty but the fact that I was wet came as news to me). I was suddenly aware of feeling anxious, uncertain, confused and no longer sure about anything. I found myself wondering if I had missed something. I asked Gemma whether I was to pretend to undress. She shook her head, and said in a quiet, reasonable tone that I had a pretty dress just like hers and that I should look after it. I was told to be worried, however. I not only felt worried but I also experienced feeling in a mess without knowing how this had happened.

In the transference I had been made aware of the shattering experience of the accident. It evoked a variety of feelings in me which clearly included an overwhelming feeling of shock. Gemma then slipped into a sticky, exciting world but a part of her ego remained in an observing role: it wasn't nice there, she said. I supported her observation by trying to fish her out and this was partially successful in that she began to symbolize her feelings through using the play dough. She carried forward this symbolic mode into the school game and my role now was to represent a part of her ego by suffering helplessly some nasty, confusing experience. I felt she had shifted from an entangled communication to a communication based on projective identification – she placed me in the same dress as herself and I felt more directly all sorts of feelings on her behalf.

Paper lampshades

The trauma of the bus accident was played out throughout the first year's work. As the year progressed, however, new material began to emerge which I felt might belong to an earlier period, though the origins of this material remained ambiguous. In the following example she was 30 minutes late for her session. She had arrived back from school in a bad mood. Upon seeing me she announced that she did not wish to go to the therapy room to make lamps, they frightened her. I suggested that we had better not make them then and reassured her it was just like any other Wednesday and that she would go back at the normal time. Once we were alone she wandered slowly to the far side of the room; she was less agitated. When she turned towards me she was holding her index finger. 'Paper, glass, lampshade,' she muttered. I gave a sympathetic 'Oh dear', and asked if that was what all the upset was about. She appeared to have hurt herself and had become very frightened of the paper in the room and of me. 'Paper lampshade,' she muttered again, sitting down next to me. I could see a small clean cut on her index finger. 'At school?' I asked. She nodded and leaning forward showed me her finger. 'Hurt,' she moaned. Picking up her tone I replied, 'Poor Gemma.'

She responded by telling me she wanted her paper bandages. I said that I thought she was telling me that she wanted me to look after her hurt and take it away. From her bent position she sat erect and in a chirpy voice said, 'Say Hello.' I said, 'Hello Gemma.' She flapped her hands and smiling returned the welcome. She then wanted me to ask her how she was, to which she replied, 'Fine.' I said I thought that she was telling me she was really pleased she had made it. She played out the hurt child and resumed her collapsed stance and staggered over to the couch with my help. The paper tubes made in a previous session were placed on her arms and legs. All the bandages had to be put on in a certain order. If this was not carried out to her satisfaction the action had to be repeated. The last bandage to go on was the stomach one. All this was reminiscent of the road accident. My task completed, I stood back.

Gemma sat up and stared unblinking at the door. She did not move a muscle. I asked what she was looking at. She shook her head and said she did not know. She held her finger up and asked for a tissue bandage. Both index fingers were then bandaged. She looked at her tissue bandage and talked of the paper lampshade – a plastic one. I was aware that, while she was clear about her meaning, I felt lost and confused.

As she continued to look at her bandaged finger, a smile crept across her face. She was slipping away, and like her I too slipped up to another gear of alertness. She gazed, fixated, at the door. I raised my voice in an effort to reach her and reminded her that she was looking at the door and the door handle. She turned and glowered at me. She slowly opened her mouth and pushed her folded tongue out. In a high-pitched voice she cried, 'Lampshade, paper, plastic, glass, hole in glass cut me.' In a firm, straightforward way I told her to put her tongue away. I pointed out that she was getting excited. I reflected that the paper had cut her, it had cut like glass but it was just paper. She put her tongue away and looked down but seconds later returned to staring at the door handle. She quickly became excited and told me that the door knob was long and had long hair. I corrected her, saying that I thought it was round. I said it did not have hair, nor was there anything exciting about it. She turned towards me and seemed desperate to communicate something. 'A long time ago there was a lampshade high up in the sky, it had long hair and came down and cut me ... in Gemma's room a long time ago. It came down and hurt me.'

She lay back on the couch, put her thumb in her mouth, and with her other hand she held her neck. She pulled her head back in an infantile way until her eyes fell on the large door knob of the cupboard behind her. She smiled. I reminded her that she was in danger of getting lost again. She laughed and remained where she was. After about a minute she sat up and held herself between the thighs. I told her to remove her hands, which she did reluctantly, but seconds later her eyes alighted on the door knob in front of her. She became distressed and said she did not like the lampshade, she was frightened and wanted to go back. I commented on how she was getting lost in the door handle and that she did not like it there. I suggested that she look away. She remained staring ahead of her. I repeated more fervently the need to look away. She turned and looked at the mantelpiece and then across to the filing cabinet.

I commented that it was difficult for her to see me. She turned and looked at me and in a shaky voice said that she was frightened. I softened my tone and explained that she was lost but that I was with her. It was almost the end of the session and, as we began to remove the bandages, she mentioned that she wanted to make a paper lampshade. I expressed some doubts at this request. She immediately became agitated, bobbing and throwing her head back, crying that she wanted to do it and take it home. I reflected that perhaps she needed to touch the paper to reassure herself that it wasn't dangerous. Having touched the paper, she again insisted that she wanted to make a lampshade. I hesitated but agreed. While I rolled a sheet of paper into a cylinder she stuck the tape across to hold it. Outside her escort was waiting. As she walked towards him she held the cylinder above her head. 'Look!' she cried. 'It's not a lampshade.'

At the beginning of the session I felt that Gemma was barely able to hold herself together. This state was reflected in how she used words, singly and spaced out, so initially they did not appear to be linked. As I helped her to sort out her thoughts, place them in time and space, she began to recover. But the lampshade and the hurt associated with it were not forgotten. It seemed that there was a drive to make the necessary link with the past. The way she moved her head and her body reminded me of a small infant. Who or what the lamp represented was not clear to me, but there was no doubting the strong link between the door, door handle and the lamp with long hair coming down and hurting her. It felt like a very early trauma, possibly involving abuse by someone opening a door and coming towards her. Whatever the meaning, it appeared to be something she had experienced passively and from which she was helpless to escape – a context similar to the one in which she had been run over by a double-decker bus. At the end of the session there was felt to be some relief and an acknowledgement that the lampshade she had made was not the one from the past. She had achieved mastery over a frightening object through actively making her own symbolic version of it.

The spider's web revisited

I have mentioned that Gemma's facial distortions reminded me of a gargoyle but to her this was her 'spider' face – it was the outward expression of her internalized spider. She told me that she believed a long time ago she was a spider. Sometimes when she withdrew she talked about going into the web – an escape from the real world, into her own sticky world. But this world was no safe psychic retreat; it was full of dangers. If she slipped too far into the web it turned against her. Her terror was that she would remain permanently caught in this world, unable to find her way back.

My second journey to this world was just before a summer break. Before leaving the waiting-room she asked for reassurance that I would be coming to see her the next day. However, for 15 minutes she ignored me. All her attention was directed towards two spiders' webs she had spotted through the window. It felt as if I did not exist for her. I commented that it seemed her world was more exciting than the two of us being together. Gemma turned and looked at me and a smile lit up her face. She said she wanted to play, and after she had been so distant her calm, friendly manner came as a surprise. The play, however, was to visit the spider's web. We agreed that if it became too much we would return together. In the game the web was sticky and I was told to cry. I tried pulling the imaginary strands away from me. 'Not like that,' she told me patiently, adding: 'Look, the web's down here.' I sat on the floor. Gemma crouched beside me. She had a fixed smile and her bulging eyes seemed to pierce me. Fright gripped me. I felt a falling sensation in the pit of my stomach. Momentarily I felt vulnerable and trapped. Gemma then pounced, wrapped her arms around my legs and said that she wanted to eat me.

I announced that this was not a nice place, that I did not want to be eaten. I said that it was horrible and that we were going back. Dutifully she held my hand and we stood up. As we cleared up she reflected that she had been a good girl. She had not thrown or destroyed any of her toys. I agreed. She then informed me that the next day was the last day of school until September. After a moment's pause she added that she would see me next week.

Alvarez (1997) states that in working with borderline children there are times when there is an imperative need, not a demand, for *someone else* to be the frightened one. By inviting me into the web Gemma was about to utilize an interpersonal context in order to let me know about aspects of her terror. In the play, itself an attempt at mastery, she would be the silent perpetrator and I would be the victim. The risk was that, as on previous occasions, she would lose herself – differentiations between self and object, animate and inanimate, would get confused. I certainly felt some of her terror but by not allowing myself to be used as an inanimate object I represented an aspect of her ego. This seemed to have helped her to recover some ego functions, to place our contact in time and space, with the result that she was able to deal with the anxiety about the coming summer holiday in much the same way as an ordinary child would.

Technical issues

Gemma's severe ego impairment (Greenspan 1989) meant that her grip on reality was a fragile one and that she could easily 'slip away' when her anxieties approached psychotic levels. These anxieties, I believe, were to do with annihilation, falling to bits, spinning away from reality, being stuck in a frightening place without a way out. Her slipping away took two different forms, however, and technically it was important to distinguish between them.

When trying to maintain contact with Gemma's psychotic state I would try to keep my communication simple, calling her name, reminding her of where she was and of my existence. I would also label emotions or actions in a straightforward way, like 'That's good', 'That's yuck', 'I'm frightened' and so on. When others were in the room I would tell her who was there. Alvarez (1992) describes how in working with borderline psychotic children a bridge is needed between reality and fantasy to help the child find the way back. My technique helped to lead Gemma back to reality and it reminded me of certain aspects of the early mother–child relationship when a mother, sensitive to her crying infant and his internal state, gently rocks and rhythmically vocalizes reassuring utterances, reminding the baby he is not alone, all is not lost.

However, there was a different atmosphere when I felt Gemma was passively losing herself in objects like a pattern or a flicking movement of a piece of string, and here I employed a more instructive method by naming reality and differentiating it from her state of mind. This method of firm but insightful management bears some resemblance to Tustin's (1988) more active approach in analytic work with autistic children, in which she advocates a more confrontative attitude towards the child's non-awareness of, or misuse of, its own body and of the therapist as a real object.

I felt this technique was all the more important on those occasions when Gemma derived a perverse pleasure from losing herself in objects or experiences. At times I felt it necessary to be quite firm about the direction she was taking, but I felt these interventions, even though they could by no means be called traditional practice, had clear therapeutic benefits because they conveyed to her that it mattered a great deal to me what she was doing to herself.

In describing her work with borderline psychotic adults, Little (1981) states: 'These patients are not able to test reality in many areas; they have to first *find* it.' In psychotic or delusional moments, she declares, reality has to be presented to the patient without the need for deduction, inference or symbol – and if reality reaches the patient's awareness then the non-psychotic part of the personality, which has been temporarily suspended, can come into play. Alvarez (1992) gives the name 'reclamation' to this activity, which she likens to the way the mother actively draws the baby back into interaction with her following periods of withdrawal. These statements come close to summarizing the work I found myself doing with Gemma, particularly during her very disturbed moments. It does not describe a technique that I considered using in advance of the treatment, but one that I came to in the course of this work, through supervision, through thinking about traumatized children, and through simply being with Gemma. I found being with her a very moving experience, and at other times quite a frightening one, but the experience was always thought-provoking – and for this thanks must go to Gemma.

Acknowledgement

Thanks must also go to Anne Alvarez for all her support and help in thinking about this case.

Chapter 8

Two forms of 'mindlessness' in the borderline psychotic child

Trevor Lubbe

I wish to illustrate through two case studies two forms of 'mindlessness' that I believe are a strong feature of the object relations pathology in children with borderline disturbance. Of the two cases I will discuss, the first has been chosen to illustrate some developments in a child with a serious mind/body problem in which his mental life was dominated by a bodily mode of primary emotional experience. The second case will describe a sophisticated defensive organization with strong borderline psychotic features in a pre-adolescent boy which required careful decoding before any shift towards more object contact and interaction could be achieved.

In recent times, developmental researchers have found a focus for core pathology in childhood around special defects in interpersonal relating and social reciprocity, which have been promulgated as defects in the child's 'theory of mind' (Hobson 1986; Baron-Cohen 1990). Along similar lines, psychoanalytic writers have cited children with borderline or 'mixed psychopathology' as displaying similar impairments (Fonagy and Higget 1990; Hobson 1993). By 'theory of mind' is meant the child's ability to 'mentalize' on a number of different representational planes: the ability to represent the personal mental world, including emotions, and the ability to impute mental states with contents to others. In addition, the problem of integrating these levels into an internal working model of self-and-object relations is also viewed as a vital developmental task awaiting completion in this group of children. Essentially, these contributions have sought to operationalize a long-standing emphasis given by psychoanalytic investigators, first to the theoretical role of object relations deficits in child psychopathology, and second to the meticulous clinical study of intersubjective psychological processes, in such a way as to make them accessible to empirical study.

While these ideas have been fruitful in conceptualizing core developmental factors, like ineffective thinking and impaired social reciprocity underlying borderline disturbance, they nonetheless require corresponding theories of 'mindlessness' if they are to address the many subtle ways in which the mind limits its own attainments – *particularly when a type of interpersonal context is being employed for this purpose*. One such psychoanalytic theory is Bion's (1962b) theory of thinking. Certain concepts within this theory, like the concept of the 'container-contained', have gained common currency in the general psychoanalytical community and beyond, but on the child front it has especially struck fertile ground in its application to the treatment of severe forms of childhood disturbance, like autism (Tustin 1972; Meltzer *et al.* 1975), severe emotional deprivation (Henry 1974) and borderline psychosis (Alvarez 1985; 1992). It is particularly Bion's developmental concepts that inform his theory as a theory of mind and a theory of 'mindlessness'.

In describing my work with these two borderline cases I shall be indicating in a practical way how some of Bion's ideas were helpful in making sense of the material. By way of a conclusion I shall be describing other clinical benefits of this theory as it applies to input and computational deficits in this group of children.

Case illustration: Mel

Mel, a boy of 8, had been placed in Social Services care periodically since the age of 5, where he was found, even at that time, to manifest a number of developmental problems like poor speech, soiling and smearing, wetting, and being prone to sudden angry outbursts – he was known to have broken a puppy's leg. Both parents had previously acknowledged their lack of care for him. His mother reported that soon after his birth she had stopped liking him when she realized she could not manage him. She had also apparently told Mel he was born a 'dead baby', but this statement was later investigated by his social worker and found 'to be false. Father had spent more time with Mel and was fond of him, but he demanded affection as a reward, and vehemently controlled him by shouting instructions. Both parents were found to be immature, chaotic and frankly neglectful of all the children in the family – a younger sister was hospitalized at 9 months because of the unhygienic conditions in the home, and an older brother of 10 had been placed on the Non-Accidental Injury register at one year of age for a fractured collar-bone and facial bruising.

When he reached the age of 7, concern was such that Mel was made a Ward of Court and placed in a children's home on a permanent basis. It was only then that the full extent of his disturbance became known to those now involved in his care. He continued to soil and play with his faeces, his enuresis spread to daytimes – even while watching TV. He attempted to start fires outside his bedroom, and he conducted himself as if impervious to pain and danger. His most disturbing symptom at this time, however, was violent masturbation which sometimes involved trying to injure his genitals by pulling or twisting. He exposed himself to staff and other residents and seemed obsessed with his penis, especially when references were made to his mother – 'My mum's got two willies,' he once said, 'my dad's and mine.' These sexual references spilled over into mealtimes, at which soft, elongated foods were referred to as 'willies'.

Mealtimes, generally, were found to be extremely anxious times for Mel. He complained of not being able to eat 'hard food', yet he also shovelled food into his mouth, swallowing it without chewing. He burped incessantly at the table, and would also pick his nose brutally. There seemed to exist no pleasure in eating at all; to observers his eating felt like a self-assault.

The repeated references by Mel to sexual matters led the professionals of the day to investigate the possibility of sexual abuse, but no conclusive evidence of this was found. Access visits by parents were promoted on a three-monthly basis.

To accompany this rather bleak and disturbing picture there were also positive reports from the children's home staff, who described Mel as an affectionate, endearing child who often surprised them with his warmth, honesty and sense of humour. His teacher found in him a passionate appetite for knowledge and skills; he loved songs and enjoyed heartily all classroom projects.

At this time Mel, aged 8, was psychiatrically assessed and diagnosed as severely emotionally deprived with 'borderline features'. He was referred to a special school for emotionally and behaviourally disturbed children, where it was decided he should undergo psychotherapy. I saw him once weekly at his school, and

I have chosen to present material from our first meetings and from two subsequent sessions, in order to illustrate the special nature of his mind/body problem, and to indicate the pathway we would take towards the development of a psychological self.

First session

The expectation and sense of high occasion invested by Mel in our first meeting became apparent the moment he entered my room. He bounded in, carrying with him a biscuit, which he placed on the table for me. He eyed the play materials and took the two cars, saying he liked the yellow one. He asked me if I had more. He sat down clutching the cars and asked again, with more urgency – 'Do you have more?' He glanced at my cupboard, twitched around on the chair, and as we sat in silence for the next few moments my cupboard and its imagined contents filled the entire room and created what felt like an excruciating barrier beyond which neither of us could move. He asked again whether I had more. Before I could reply, he switched his attention to the biscuit, touching it nervously. Then he stood up, hovered over it, giggled, and in no time at all, the biscuit had come to replace my cupboard as an apparent source of extreme existential agony for him.

He offered it to me again, then withdrew it, laughing. Then he broke off a small piece and ate it. This was followed by more giggles and more nibbles from the biscuit until, with a triumphant flourish, he declared, 'It's all gone!' I felt strangely relieved, and thought that he must be showing me something of an experience of being offered something only to see it vanish or taken away, bit by bit. I put this to him, saying that if a boy felt he'd been given something nice, only to see it taken away, he would certainly find it important to know whether there was more. I then thought it immediately necessary to explain the purpose of our meetings, and I outlined the setting and the practical arrangements.

Mel listened intently to what I had to say, but suddenly, as if permission had been given, he grabbed the boy doll, put both its feet into his mouth and bit hard. He then took the scissors and tried to cut them off. I cautioned him and, instead, he put one of the cars into his mouth and with all his might he bit off one of the wheels. Then he became very tense, giggled, and poked his finger up the girl doll's dress, twisting her legs.

I spoke about his showing me a very hard biting mouth that could break things off. He said there was a spider once, with long legs and teeth, that could bite. He went to the mirror and with a black pen scribbled on his front teeth. Then he approached me menacingly, open-mouthed. I responded by saying that *he* was now being a spider-boy with a hard, biting mouth who could frighten people by wanting to gobble everything up. He touched his genitals and said he had to go to the toilet. I waited for him and after a few minutes I went out and found him lolling about in the corridor. I took him by the hand and led him back to the room, where he seemed calmer. He sat on the floor playing with the cars but this play took on a desultory, lifeless quality. I said the spider-boy had now stopped wanting to bite and gobble everything up, but this had left him flat and disappointed. He looked up at me – 'Can I take these cars with me?' The school bell suddenly rang and he bounded out, leaving the cars.

While I could not fail to be impressed by Mel's openness and directness in this our first meeting, by his 'diving straight in' so to speak, and treating me like a new positive object, and while I felt that some contact between us had been made, I was nevertheless left uneasy about the precocious nature of this contact and how this may have drawn me into 'diving in' too soon with some of my comments. I was aware, for instance, of how he touched his genitals when I addressed his menacing mouth, and this drew my immediate attention to the concreteness of his experiences. I was struck, I suppose, by his defensive deficiency, by his vulnerability as a consequence of being so open and appearing to have no natural barrier or boundary between impulses directed at him from without and within. I was reminded of Anna Freud's caveat about the relative ease with which interpretations can be made with children in whom id content is relatively unchecked (1965: 232).

I was also left in no doubt about my own vulnerability in terms of what a volatile and demanding therapy this might prove. But Mel himself seemed unconsciously aware of this factor: the high tension in the room around 'more' toys and the interactions around the biscuit reflected, I felt, a communication about supplies – whether there *were* enough supplies, and whether these supplies might survive the oral destructive maraudings of a ravenous little spider-boy. I wondered too about the impact of these impulses upon his self- and object-representations, and whether the 'deadness' towards the end of the session reflected a despairing conviction that in the face of such violent impulses, which are capable of sweeping all before them, it would not be possible for any conception of a 'good' object to prevail. Having been swept up in the drama of our opening encounter I had not, as yet, addressed in my mind how his behaviour reflected his real-life circumstances.

Sessions 2–4

Mel missed the next session because of illness so I offered a rearranged time later on in the week. He arrived for this session carrying a yellow car of his own which he propelled across the threshold of my door, explaining that this was a 'special' car. I welcomed the new car inside, saying, 'This is a special car coming at a special time.' He chuckled and came in, and immediately set up the floor-rug into a ramp from which the cars were rolled to see whether they could go down 'smooth'. Gradually a ridge formed itself across the centre of the rug which interfered with the smooth flow of the cars. Mel called this ridge a 'lump' and began pushing the cars violently into it to get it out of the way. I said he wanted things to come and go smoothly but hard lumps kept getting in the way.

He replied that he had had a lump in his throat since our last meeting – that's why he couldn't come to see me earlier in the week. I talked about different kinds of lumps in the throat – some to do with a sore throat and some to do with being upset. He immediately touched his genitals and moved the cars to the table, where he made them drop off one by one. These were 'crashes', he claimed, and he developed this game using the doll family. Each family member was made to cling onto another's shoulders until it fell to the floor. 'Hang on! Hang on!' they cried, but to no avail.

This game was repeated over and over again, and a dog was placed below to attack the last member to fall – the mother doll. She called out to be rescued but her fate was sealed. Again I had a strong sense of Mel's vulnerability as to the impact of what I might say about this game, but I felt I had seen enough and could not remain silent. I said, 'This is your family, and what if they are in some danger? You worry sometimes about something happening to them and you won't be able to help.' He blinked and swallowed hard, and he grabbed all the wild animals to make them attack the mother doll, ripping her clothes. I lowered my voice and said this game was showing me some of his feelings about his absent family, strong feelings, which perhaps felt like lumps inside him. Astonishingly, he took the Sellotape and devised a 'bridge' from the floor to the bookshelf so that the boy doll could be rescued. But his respite was brief: the boy now found himself alone on the shelf as a spider approached. I said it was the boy who was now in danger and there seemed no way his family could reach and help him.

At the start of the next session Mel refused to enter the room. 'No way! No way I'm coming in here!' he bellowed from the corridor. I left the door ajar, and after appearing and disappearing several times from the entrance, he eventually came in, carrying a collection of cars from his classroom. He immediately set up the ramp again, angrily rolling two cars down to cause a crash. The cars were then backed into one another, causing them to be knocked across the room. I said the cars were now like lumps getting in one another's way. He collected the doll family and dangled them again from the table, letting them drop. This time the grandparent dolls were included, with the grandfather doll coming in for particularly harsh treatment – his coat was torn off and he was dropped from a greater height.

I said the grandfather doll stood for me, and that he was angry with me because when my door was shut that felt like 'no way' he could come inside to get his therapy cars. He became very tense and dropped the little girl doll into the wastepaper bin, farting unexpectedly. He laughed and exclaimed, 'It's like poohs!' Then all the dolls were dropped into the bin, the grandfather doll included. I said he was now showing me what it felt like to be treated like poohs. He emptied the bin and flung all its contents at me. Then he tried to bite the grandmother doll, but stopped and tore her dress off instead. I said, without thinking, 'She's naked now, she's got no protection.' He quickly stopped and moved to cutting the table with the scissors, then the ruler, and in the end I had to retrieve the dangerous scissors. He now pelted me with lumps of Plasticine, calling me 'lucky' when I avoided being hit. 'I'm taking all the cars,' he cried, and retreated to a corner of the room.

I surveyed the total chaos in the room. I found myself gathering up strewn pieces of Plasticine from the floor, which seemed to go in tandem with collecting my thoughts. Mel stayed in the corner, playing quietly. I sat down and suddenly felt overcome with a great sadness. This boy must feel he has lost everything, I thought. Notwithstanding his terrible past and the recorded neglect by his parents, he must feel that his whole world is in pieces. And it must also seem to him as if no living authority could address his situation in a meaningful way. I recalled that throughout the many case discussions and assessments I had read about this boy there had been no reference made to his actual loss of a family, and the violent, castrating way in which this appears to have been experienced by him. I chided myself for being so direct in my interpretations and questioned whether my therapeutic approach, and the once-weekly regime, might not traumatize him further. We ended with all the cars, except the yellow one, being taken back to the classroom.

The following session was delayed because of strike action by teachers at the school, which meant another session had to be rearranged later in the week. Mel made a disgruntled entrance, carrying with him a toy motorbike with a little boy rider. He called me a 'shit' and sat down to dismantle the toy, taking the boy off his bike, taking his helmet off, removing his gloves and his windshield. He said this boy had hurt his knee, he had fallen down and 'jumped out of his skin'. I asked why there was such a cross voice today and he replied, 'Because you've done a big shit. What colour is your shit?' he asked defiantly. 'Is it green?'

I knew he had shown me a bike-boy stripped of his defences, but I wanted to answer his question. I said perhaps green was a bad colour today because Ms Greenson (his teacher) and I had not been available to him because the school had been shut for two days. He did not react but made the motorbike growl instead, but his subsequent play again began to take on an empty, lifeless feel. Gradually, however, the boy rider was re-equipped, put back onto his bike and made to skid around the table, closer and closer to the edge. I said, 'This boy has got his skin back but he may yet be in danger.' Predictably, the bike was made to topple on to the floor. The doll family then joined in, not to help, but to push the boy aside and take over the bike. The mother drove with the father on her shoulders, and the other children clutching his back. I asked what was going on and he replied, 'Oodles of noodles of cuddles of kisses.' Then, excitedly, he made all the family members pile violently on top of one another and do 'exercises' which resembled indiscriminate sexual activity.

I spoke firmly and said this was a jumble, and that there was a jumble in his mind every time he had strong feelings inside. The strong feelings today, I said, were called hurt and angry; he was hurt and angry with Ms Greenson and me for not being there for him earlier on in the week, so in his mind he'd made us into a nasty sex-exercising couple making pooh babies. He laughed and grabbed the dolls and smelled their genitals. 'They're OK,' he declared. For the first time he helped pack away at the end of the session.

Comment

Except for this last exchange, what comes across so vividly in these opening sessions is the extent to which practically all forms of emotionality are experienced by Mel in a very concrete way. Obviously there are many aspects of this boy's past experiences that have not been mentalized owing to their having retained a degree of encapsulated rawness which is liable to be triggered off when any reference to his inner world is made. Again, authors like Eckstein and Wallerstein (1954) have suggested we avoid 'trigger language' in areas where the child appears vulnerable. Yet one area of rawness needs to be separated from another, and I believed a very specific area of rawness, hitherto passed over, had presented itself for consideration during our opening interactions and my comments. This was Mel's experience of loss and violent abandonment: the loss by Mel of a family life, however chaotic or neglectful, and his sense of having been cruelly abandoned. From this viewpoint the desultory play suggested an underlying bereavement and depression. This had emerged mainly through his sensitivity and hurt about the cars – of my giving them to him but then taking them away – and the missed session. Yet the appearance of another yellow car in session 3 suggested to me a degree of psychological-mindedness (object constancy) in retaining a link between the sessions, notwithstanding the violent play that followed.

There are many other themes that merit discussion but I would like to keep the focus on the issue of 'mindlessness'. In Mel's case this is manifested in his visceral experience of feeling states, as exemplified in the way he perceives all forms of satisfaction and dissatisfaction to involve 'lumps'. Whether these lumps refer to 'hard food', or to lumps in the throat that cause him to miss school, or lumps in the carpet which obstruct the flow of cars, or to angry lumps in his bottom, or indeed to verbal lumps his therapist is asking him to consider – they describe emotional data and experiences that have not been fully mentalized (Fonagy 1991). They have yet to obtain a psychological value or meaning by virtue of being sufficiently privileged in the mind of the object, failing which they cannot serve as a restraint to action or reaction, nor can they be represented other than in bodily terms and thereby be subject to bodily pathways of disburdenment. Mel's use of the synthetic function is limited, and he is operating at what Bion (1962b) called a 'proto-mental' level, where 'thinking' operates on the same model as motor discharge – to get rid of painful contents rather than modify them.

The overly sexualized nature of Mel's concretizations certainly requires serious comment. Some authors have noted in their work the high incidence of precocity in the way, for example, phallic or genital elements become interwoven with oral elements (Rosenfeld and Sprince 1963), or the way anal and genital preoccupations were found as related themes (Szur 1983). Mel's own psychosexual 'jumble' of oral, phallic and genital themes is conveyed in his motorbike play and in his description of the doll family's engagement in 'oodles of noodles of cuddles of kisses', which quickly becomes eroticized. His analization of the breast, which is evident from his treatment of soft, elongated food, is also an index of the phase confusion of his libidinal development. Another way of stating this is to say that solutions for unresolved oral conflicts may be sought at anal or phallic levels, and if these oral conflicts are centred on sadistic or cannibalistic issues then their anal or phallic expressions are all the more likely to contain violent or brutal features.

I will now present some material from six months into the therapy to show the beginnings of a mentalizing process with respect to Mel's predominantly bodily mode of experience.

Mel had visited my room earlier in the day, knocking at my door, and I had to remind him that his session was later in the afternoon. Unknown to me this visit had followed a classroom incident in which he had swallowed a small iron ball-bearing, causing great alarm and necessitating a trip to the local hospital for an X-ray. He returned to school that afternoon in time for his session and brought with him a large Lego battleship adorned with two toy figures armed with guns. He told me this toy belonged to Jim, another boy in his class, and he reassured me he was not going to 'mash it up'. He dismantled a small section of the ship, but put it back together again, and told me that he had missed school lunch that day because he'd been taken out by his teacher. He then explained that he'd been to the doctor because he'd swallowed a ball-bearing. 'You know, those round things – they're hard!'

I said this must have been frightening for him, and I wondered whether that was why he had called on me earlier in the day. He stood up and said he wanted to go to the toilet. I said he seemed frightened now, thinking about what had happened to him. He squatted on the floor and said he was going to do a big shit. I took his hand and led him to the toilet, where, inside, I heard him straining and muttering the word 'ball-bearing' to himself. Eventually he came out and told me the word 'ball-bearing' was a hard word to say. On our return to the room we passed a female teacher and Mel pulled a face and began to walk in a disjointed way. 'I'm handicapped!' he screeched. As we entered the room he turned to me and said triumphantly, 'That frightened her!'

Immediately he took apart the battleship, dismantling it almost completely. This tested me and I wanted to stop him. I said he was now mashing up Jim's battleship, taking it apart, in the same way as he'd made himself fall apart in the corridor. He laughed but carried on. I suggested that going to the toilet had not worked in getting rid of his frightened feelings about the ball-bearing, so he needed to put those frightened feelings outside, into the teacher in the corridor and into me, to see if we could mash them up for him.

He pushed the Lego to one side and turned his attention to a mask from the previous session. This mask had been used to disguise some curious peering at me for most of that session, which I had not properly understood. He now scolded me for not letting him take it home. 'You're such an egghead,' he said. Then he wanted to draw, and searched the room for a subject.

Eventually his eyes settled upon me and he told me to keep still. 'And keep your hand under your chin.' He then drew, to my great surprise, an extremely delicate head-and-shoulders portrait of me. As he traced my features with his gaze, his eyes widened and he gave me a warm, radiant smile. A look of glowing appreciation also came into his expression as he studied me. I was deeply touched and could not myself resist a smile. 'Keep still,' he said, and he struggled for some time to get my arm and hand correctly positioned under my chin. 'That's your thinking position,' he said.

Comment

Better, I think, to call a ball-bearing a 'hard' word to say than to swallow one as an attempt to digest a frightening experience. Better still to search out your 'egg-head' therapist for the purposes of externalizing 'lumps', so that they may at least be given the opportunity to be mashed up or 'smoothed'. At least the feeding function in this material appears momentarily to be uncontaminated by phallic and anal themes.

My early countertransference feelings around Mel's psychological nakedness, his lack of a protective or filtering mechanism for emotional stimuli, and his vulnerability to 'trigger language', particularly by an overzealous therapist, occupied my thinking throughout this therapy, which lasted three years. Obviously this lack reflected the fragile and disorganized state of his ego, where a physical self clearly took precedence over a psychological self, but in my work I had to balance this concern with another strong impression, namely, that certain ego functions were sufficiently intact to allow me to give names to those feelings centred on his real-life situation. Of course, an appalling internal reality had to be faced too, and my efforts here led initially to strong reactions, but I felt encouraged by the way in which my interventions in this direction led to clear themes emerging, like the theme of 'lumps'.

As I have mentioned, these 'lumps' referred to a legacy of unmentalized painful emotions, particularly around loss and rejection, that could find expression only in concretizations, self-destructiveness and acting-out. This was evidence to me of a damaged core, of a damaged psychic apparatus which could not carry through its representational and transformational tasks in the service of integration.

Second case illustration: Brian

Brian, a boy of 14, had previously received one year of weekly psychotherapy on an outpatient basis before transferring to me when his therapist left. He had been a pupil at a local special school for emotionally disturbed children since the age of 6, and was described to me by his teachers as a 'strange' boy who daydreamed a lot, and spent most of his school day drifting around or burrowing away at random activities without producing much in the way of work.

History

Brian was born to very young, runaway parents who physically abused and neglected him when he was 2 months old during a period of upheaval and stress in their relationship. He was hospitalized with a broken leg, cracked ribs, and a mark on his forehead consistent with a burn. His mother received a custodial sentence during which time she was treated for depression. After a year-long separation, the family were reunited, though Brian remained on a supervision care order until the age of 5.

At the time of going into care, Brian was described as an agitated, hard-to-hold baby who slept and ate poorly and who provoked firm, sometimes aggressive handling. As a young child attending nursery, he was described as an overactive, chaotic little boy, who suffered from chronic colds and night-time terrors, and was generally delayed in his attainments. Subsequent to his admission to school, the reports continued of an overactive, impulsive child, who appeared confused and disorganized in his activities, and whose contact with other children was characterized by fear or excessive clinginess.

There then followed, with the help of substantial input from his school, a period of remarkable progress in Brian's ego development which enabled him to make considerable gains in his speech and written work. However, in his social contact with teachers and fellow pupils, the picture persisted of a chaotic boy, who 'bounced' off those around him, and inevitably ended up isolated in his own private world of bizarre noises and gestures culled from television programmes.

When I first met Brian's parents they were frankly opposed to further therapy. I sensed in them an acute sensitivity regarding their past abuse of their son, around which they had constructed an elaborate myth centred on damage done to Brian by outsiders. Their distress about Brian's development, however, was palpable; they openly despaired about what they described as his laziness and forgetfulness and their chronic inability to understand him.

One comment of theirs struck a note of recognition in me with regard to my diagnostic thinking. They spoke about Brian's virtuosity in grasping the ins and outs of spaceship technology, but in the same sentence they mentioned his frequent disappearances – 'getting lost' on his way home from the shops. After further discussion they agreed to a continuation of once-weekly psychotherapy in his school setting.

I shall be discussing details of the first six months of Brian's therapy, which was concluded after 18 months when he completed school.

First impressions

When I met Brian for the first time, he told me gravely that he liked talking in the mornings but wasn't much good in the afternoons. He announced that he had just taken a weekend job at a local hospital as a doorman, a job given to him following an incident in which he had rescued a young woman who had become trapped in the revolving doors at the hospital entrance. 'Imagine', he said portentously, 'if this had been someone suffering from a heart attack? I help others if they help me.'

These opening remarks sounded convincing enough, but it soon became apparent that I had to treat them not as 'truths' but as raw material which had to be deciphered. In the course of our first session, therefore, the following 'facts' were established: Brian had seen his previous therapist, a young woman, at this hospital in the mornings. He missed his therapist terribly, and missed his sessions too – which had been literally life-saving to him. He often found himself wandering past the hospital at weekends, and he said he felt hurt, outraged, 'going around in circles' since these sessions had stopped.

Once we had established this line of contact via my deciphering, Brian relaxed visibly and indicated that he was pleased to come to my room. He said he knew by heart all the rooms in the school and complimented himself on his good memory. When he was 5 years old, he recalled, he was standing in a field with his parents when a glider passed overhead: 'At first it was faint, but it grew louder and louder and I was frightened.' He then recalled being at the seaside at the age of 2, again with his parents, standing at the water's edge, watching it encroach and being unable to move. Quickly, however, he changed tack and asked me if I had a pet cat. His own cat, he explained, liked to snuggle up to him when it wanted feeding. 'I feed him in the mornings, the afternoons, and the evenings, and let him snooze on my bed.'

I commented on this considerate, caring attitude, and wondered whether that was the reason he questioned me about having a cat, that is, to check what my caring attitude might be in the light of my offering myself as his new therapist. He stared at me and said, 'How do you know my code?' Then, switching again, he commented on my radiator, wondering how hot it might get in this room. At home, he said, they had installed new radiators which meant he now had two heaters in his bedroom. 'I have to turn one down if it gets too hot,' he explained. I smiled and said (thinking this was a reference to changing therapists) that perhaps two heaters meant he had a spare one if something went wrong.

He agreed, and turned his attention to the drawing materials, suggesting he'd like to write his name on a book, 'in pencil, if you don't mind'. I said that, while it might be reassuring to him if I understood his code, I could also understand it if he was uncertain about me, worried, on the one hand, about whether I was the reliable sort and might stick around for him, and worried, on the other hand, about things getting too intense. 'You know this teacher's strike that's on the go next week?' he broke in. 'Well, one thing I can't understand – is it just at this school or is it all over the world?' I felt adroitly deflected, and realized that Brian's psychological 'thermostat' (Eckstein and Wallerstein 1954) had kicked in to control the situation. We made arrangements for our weekly meetings on Wednesday afternoons, and Brian tidied the desk before leaving. 'See you next Thursday,' he said cheerfully as he closed the door.

Comment

What struck me about this opening session was how much the question of contact – of how it is made, sustained or broken – was at the centre of Brian's communications. The dependency of ego structure in borderline cases upon object contact has been well documented by previous authors (Eckstein 1966). A number of powerful anxieties surrounding contact were also greatly in evidence, and I sought clarification of those in subsequent sessions. I understood the story about becoming a doorman at the hospital he had attended previously for therapy as a powerful phantasy being expressed through projective identification. All his feelings of panic, bewilderment, loss and helplessness concerning the ending of his sessions have been projected into the young woman going through the hospital door in order that he, in action, could identify himself with a helping, benevolent doorman who, like all good cat lovers (and all good therapists), are at their posts morning, noon and night to ensure a total service. The anger towards those who set themselves up as carers, but who inevitably let you down, is clearly present in this phantasy, as is the resulting sense of a confusion between reality and phantasy. The fact that little or nothing of the report had taken place in reality underlined its status as a powerful, omnipotent phantasy. His recollections of the scene on the beach and the scene in the field, however, I understood not as phantasies but more in the nature of screen memories that referred to his early lived experience of abuse and subsequent removal from his parents. Certainly a strong impression of being unsafe in the presence of good objects is poignantly conveyed in these reports.

In the next session Brian drew a picture of a car with a prominent back wheel and an exhaust pipe emitting fumes. He reported that he'd been reading a story about smoke spreading across the country, and that a man who had been feeding sheep had been killed. 'I assure you, though,' he said directly to me, 'Michael Knight [a TV character] is not programmed to kill.'

I suggested the drawing expressed his worry about our contact and whether it would be something like a feed or something more dangerous. He promptly wrote the date at the top of the picture as 'FRI-day' and mumbled, 'That's the day you *fry*, boy.' I said his worry was that if we made contact someone might get burned or poisoned. 'Dead right!' he retorted. Perhaps to be 'right' then, I said, to be able to understand his code, would give us access to his real feelings, but this might be very frightening for him.

At this very early stage in our contact I could see that we were up against several prominent anxieties with respect to the approach by an object towards Brian, and the prospect of possible contact with it: (i) that he might be attacked, (ii) that he might attack and possibly destroy the object, (iii) that he might as a consequence lose his object and find himself alone, disconnected and filled with dread.

Throughout the literature on the borderline child it has often been noted that an acute concern for the object's loss, with consequent feelings of guilt and grief, is a typical feature of the anxiety states belonging to this group of children (Mahler 1971; Masterson 1972; Vela *et al*. 1983). Frijling-Schreuder (1969) aptly likens this group to toddlers whose mothers are permanently out of the room. In Kleinian terminology, the descriptive lack of object constancy and the sense of embattled isolation which this leads to is attributed dynamically to a chronic interplay between persecutory and depressive anxieties (Rey 1979; Steiner 1979).

At this early point I had some sense that, by living in a coded world, a world of evasion of real contact and real emotional communication, Brian could to some extent mitigate the upsurge of persecutory and depressive anxieties associated with his felt dealings and interactions with others. The coded world was created mainly through phantasies of projective identification which placed him at the 'borders' of interpersonal contact, but at a price paid in terms of restricted emotional development. During the next sequence of sessions these forms of anxiety around contact were more prevalent, requiring from me further attempts to rein them in and possibly transform them through continued deciphering. I would like to illustrate a certain development in the material, and a certain development towards mindfulness, by referring specifically to Brian's drawings during these sessions.

The drawing in Figure 1 depicts a space battleship firing at a planet upon which it proposed to land, but which had unexpectedly revealed its hostile intentions. This drawing followed Brian's late arrival for his session, to which he had brought a geometry kit. He began working quietly on his own, accompanying himself with a song: 'I lost my heart to a starship trooper, flashing lights in hyperspace.' I had been silent so far and he looked up at me and asked if I was still talking to him. I replied that I thought the planet in the picture stood for my room, where he had intended to land today, but his late arrival and his asking me whether I was still talking to him suggested that he was unsure as to what kind of reception he'd receive today, friendly or unfriendly.

He warmed to this line of investigation and began another drawing (Fig. 2) of a top-elevation view of my room. He continued with his song and looked up at the skylight saying, 'It's open today.' (In fact it was closed.) 'Mmm, smells good,' he added, rocking back and forth on his chair. I said he was looking for a safe place to land here with me, a smell-good place, that was steady and would not rock around under his feet. 'Rock around

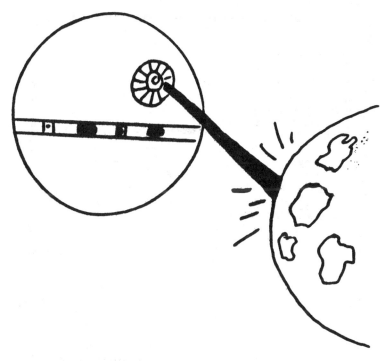

Fig. 1

the clock!' he screeched, gyrating on the chair in what seemed to me like a masturbatory movement. Then he suddenly sobered up, a serious expression came over him, and he resumed his song in a much sadder key: 'I lost my heart to a starship trooper, flashing lights in hyperspace.'

At the start of the next session Brian entered the room with a loud bang on the door and greeted me with a 'Hello–goodbye'. He had returned with his geometry kit, but left it to one side and, free-hand, drew a picture of a car from the 'top elevation' (Fig. 3). This car included two head-rests, safety belts and an aerial. The belts, he said, could be made to 'connect-off'. He then produced an odd whining noise which sounded like someone tuning into a radio station – 'Come in, come in – are you receiving me?'

I commented on the car's safety features and suggested that the presence of an aerial implied that some contact and communication was possible. But I also drew attention to his 'Hello–goodbye'

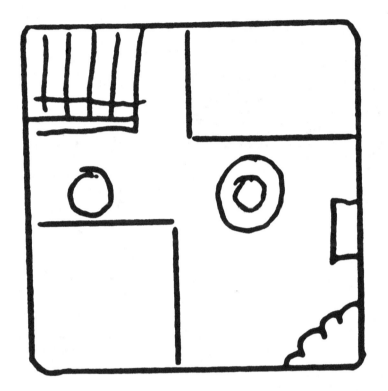

Fig. 2

form of entry into the room, and wondered whether this reflected his uncertainty about coming, which meant he would have to be ready to 'connect-off' if necessary.

He studied the interior of my room for the first time, and with the aid of a ruler he drew two versions of my cupboard – a 'front-elevation' view and a 'top-elevation' view (Figs 4 and 5). Inside the 'top-elevation' figure he drew a square which represented his tray of materials inside my cupboard.

While he drew, he explained that his teacher had told him to use his imagination, but the trouble was, he couldn't control his imagination. On the other hand, he continued, he had a cousin who could control his imagination. He reported that he had visited this cousin, a boy of his own age, during the holidays but that this boy had not bothered to phone or keep in touch with him.

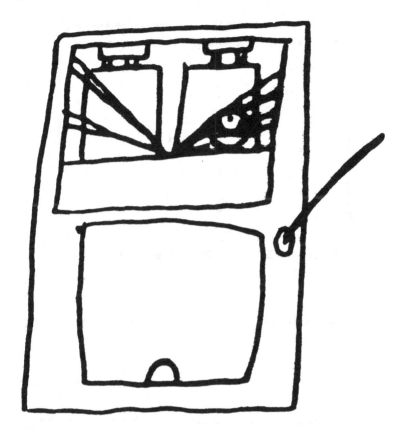

Fig. 3

He suddenly got up and paced the room in great annoyance, moving suddenly towards the door as if to go out. I jumped up and said I didn't want him to leave, which seemed to jar him out of his state of agitation, and he sat down timidly on one of the chairs. I said he had shown me today through his drawings of the car and the cupboard that he had a good idea of what an inside place looked like, an inside place like an imagination, where things could be kept and perhaps thought about. He appeared calmer but continued to grumble on about his cousin. I suggested that sometimes hurt and angry thoughts arose in his imagination too, which caused him to 'connect-off' with people.

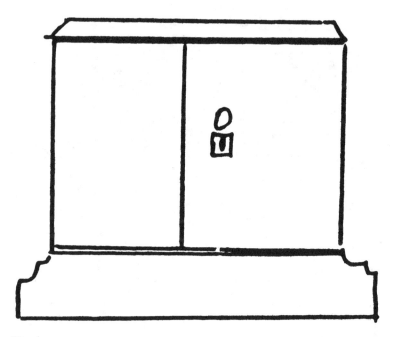

Fig. 4

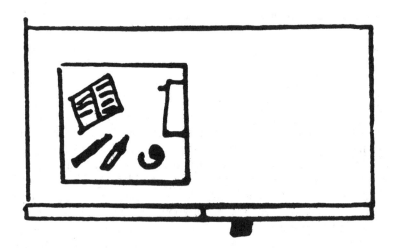

Fig. 5

The next session produced a dramatic portrait of a fierce-looking figure from a computer game (Fig. 6). Right in the belly of this figure was a box-shaped structure called a 'deactivation chamber' whose job it was to deactivate 'powerful incoming signals'. I suggested this figure represented the pushy therapist of the previous session who had said 'no' to his leaving the room. I said perhaps this had frightened him and had also made him angry, but the idea of a 'deactivation chamber' made it possible for powerful and angry feelings to be made less powerful and angry. Brian agreed and drew a picture of an eye (Fig. 7) with the title, 'For your eyes only'. He sang the James Bond theme tune and said his favourite group was called Madness. I suggested there was a fear of looking inside things in case something mad was discovered.

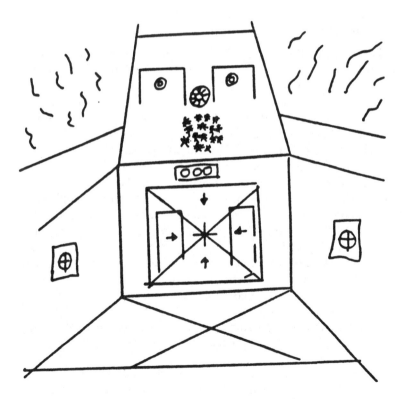

Fig. 6

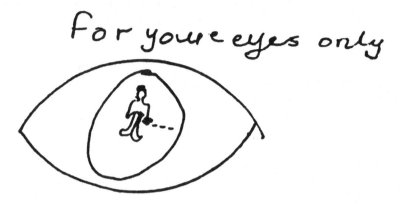

Fig. 7

Commentary

The impact of this sequence of sessions has been to allow three related ideas to unfold in the therapy: the idea of a 'landing platform' and the idea of an 'inside space' with its function as a 'deactivation chamber', all of which, I believe, are references to mental functions, and have features in common with Bion's concept of the 'container-contained'.

The 'landing platform' represents a surface capable of some measure of steadfastness, resilience and safety when faced with Brian's desperate but wavering search for contact with his object. The risk of a crash-landing is high (entering with a bang), as is the likelihood of a hostile reception (the planet repelling invaders), hence the need for a 'connect-off' approach which typically leaves Brian hovering. He is hovering on the cusp between object cathexis and identification (Rosenfeld and Sprince 1963). The 'landing platform' also has some features in common with a two-dimensional view of objects described by Meltzer *et al.* (1975) in relation to childhood autism, in so far as the surfaces of objects are experienced as inseparable from their sensual qualities (smells good), and there is little sense of an internal space into which things can fit.

The idea of an 'inside space' marks the beginnings of a 'container' in Bion's sense – a place, as opposed to a surface, for putting things into. At this point Brian refers to his imagination, but we observe that this imagination can be used as a means of approaching his object as well as a means of propelling him backwards into outer space. The tricky task for the therapist is to know when the developmental possibilities of an 'inside space' are being used as an apparatus for psychic work, or when it is being used in reverse for defensive purposes (Alvarez 1992: 117).

With the emergence of the notion of a 'deactivation chamber', a shift is evident from a sensation-dominated experience of objects to a view of the object as capable of apprehending, looking inside and deciphering powerful emotional signals. Implicit in this shift is the potential in the self for moderating as opposed to evading emotions. In other words, an apparatus for thinking and remembering was now emerging based upon the functions of a 'deactivation chamber' which could allow for certain thoughts and emotions, previously inadmissible to consciousness, to find expression. Just to what purpose this apparatus would now be put I had no way of knowing at this point, even though there were clear indications from Brian's very first sessions of what this might be.

Further clinical material

The following session comes from the seventh month of therapy. Brian had missed a session (and a school outing) because of illness, and he returned complaining bitterly that no one really cared about him or looked after him properly. He announced that he was going to run away from home, to live with his cousin, who really appreciated and understood him. He would send his cousin a postcard informing him of this plan, but he would send the card ahead, anonymously, to see whether his handwriting would be recognized. In a sarcastic tone he enquired whether I had anything to say about this plan.

I said he knew perfectly well I'd be interested in such a plan, but it sounded as if my interest would arrive too late. He huffed and puffed, and I spoke to him about how terrible it must have been for him last week, being ill, being at home alone with his parents at work, without school, without his sessions, and I wondered whether a part of him was in great need of being helped and understood today. He gave a hollow, dismissive laugh, and I said straightforwardly that I believed there was another part of him that sounded too angry to do any kind of wanting, and that this part usually made it jolly difficult for others to reach him and help him.

He tore up an envelope he was making, suggesting the paper was no good. I felt some rising impatience and said, 'I think this part of you that sometimes hates wanting and needing seems to believe that no one is really good enough to look after you.'

He sank in his chair and became so floppy that he decided to lie down on the soft chairs. He said this was 'true'; he often didn't tell me what was going on in his life, or what had happened to him in the past. He said with great feeling that as a baby he had been in an accident. He'd been left in the back seat of a car and someone had broken in and damaged his ribs and legs. He said he couldn't understand how anyone could do such a thing, or how such a thing could be allowed. He closed his eyes and said the incident had been so shocking there had been an item on television about it. 'I just can't believe how such a thing could happen.' After a pause he said it felt peculiar lying on the chairs, it was like being in a cot, like being reborn. 'Everyone should get reborn every five years,' he said.

The atmosphere in the room was extremely serious and infused with pain. I had no idea of what to make of this last statement, except that it must form part of Brian's grappling in the moment with the 'unthought known' (Bolas 1991) aspects of his abuse as a baby. There was little I could say and time passed until the end of the session. He got up to leave but mentioned at the door that his birthday was the following week, and he asked whether his session fell on that day. We checked the dates but they didn't coincide, to which he responded with a terrific show of despair and angry resignation – 'Oh well, it just goes to show, doesn't it?' He shot out of the room and I felt shot through with a pang of guilt.

Later on, when I had time to recover my feelings and review the session, I thought his comments about rebirth were a sign of hopefulness, a statement that if the damage of the past could be faced, whether as myth or as truth, then things could be started over. My confronting him about his mistrust and repudiation of good-enough objects seemed to go to the heart of his acute disbelief in the trustworthiness of objects which, of course, has been so evident by his retreat from, and deep anxieties about, contact with others. It was this internal situation that had to be further modified in the next phase of therapy.

Commentary

Receiving a projection of guilt from Brian after six months of therapy, unexpected though this was for the therapist, felt like a great advance from my usual experience in the room of having continually to cast forth a mind-net in the hope of luring parts of this boy's emotional intelligence from its migration through deep space. Literally, the therapist had to make it worth while for Brian to engage in human contact of a non-peremptory nature, and sometimes this needed to be done quite assertively.

The use of projection was therefore an important step forward from Brian's characteristic 'hovering' between mental states, his occupying a sort of no man's land in respect of feelings, or else burying his feelings in 'code'. This was a child who either made no impression on others, who was easily forgotten or left to busy himself in his own private world, or who made his presence known through abrasive collisions or excessive clinginess. What I needed to understand, however, was that these strategies were part of Brian's defensive wrapping which protected him, and his objects, from the full impact of emotional contact. In a later session, when discussing his anger, Brian stated: 'There are two types of rebellion, rebellion of the good, and rebellion of the bad,' which I understood as a statement about his fear and mistrust of all forms of emotion.

Brian never encountered the 'absolute' truth of his abuse by his parents during this therapy – but this was not a therapeutic goal. Instead, his struggle became centred on the idea of an abused and damaged part of himself, which at first he ridiculed and hated, and then was able to treat with some measure of concern and compassion. This struggle, I believe, involved a kind of 'knowing' the truth which helped to lessen the grip of a defensive organization upon his personality, and allowed some forward movement.

I would like to illustrate this struggle by quoting from our final session. Brian came in and immediately drew attention to a mark on the table, saying it reminded him of Halley's Comet. 'I'll never be the same as Sean [a classmate], you know,' he complained. 'He's got a job at McDonald's – fuck, I'm so thick.' He wrote his name on his wrist and said, 'This is the sign of death.' Then he took his pulse and lay down on the chairs. I felt a sudden panic for his safety, and recalled the scenario he presented at our first meeting of the woman in panic, trying to get through the hospital doors. I said his thoughts had turned to our ending and to how he might manage without therapy, and that these were panicky thoughts. Perhaps he also wondered, I added, whether he could return here (Halley's Comet) to visit once he left school.

'I have to fight for my own life now,' he replied crossly. 'You know that bomber-jacket I got for Christmas – perhaps I'll get it bullet-proofed.' Then he laughed, sat up and reflected, 'Now *that's* thick.' There was a pause and he said, 'Maybe I'll just go slowly at first. My dad has offered me a job on his team, but that's only next year. Anyway, these Yanks – they're such show-offs with their War of Independence!'

One final comment on Brian's progress while he was in therapy. He showed considerable improvement in his academic performance at school; he passed three final school exams and, given his profound attachment to his school, his final weeks there went off successfully. He attended the final school assembly, brought presents for his teachers, and read out a poem entitled 'Ten Years in One School'. In saying his goodbyes, however, he gave a confused and grandiose account of a recent job interview.

Conclusion

The child in whom a borderline symptom profile is salient may be in no position routinely to utilize psychotherapy, since his inner world may be so disorganized that thoughts and emotions may have no obvious apparatus for their expression, and object relations may lack the kind of 'linking' to others which allows communication to take place. Both these deficiencies may be portrayed as variations of 'mindlessness'. In these circumstances the clinician requires a model to help distinguish one level of psychological abstraction from another, one level of psychological reality from another, as well as some means of exploring the necessary preconditions for mental life itself.

There are several features of Bion's theory of thinking which I believe privilege its status as a coherent theory of 'mindlessness': (i) the theory includes subsidiary concepts, like alpha function and beta elements, which address developmental as well as repetition compulsion elements at the perceptual, pre-linguistic and metacognitive stages in the development of thought, e.g. the progression from pre-conception to conception, the transmuting of bodily modes of primary experience into mental modes of experience; (ii) the theory relates mental growth to emotional conditions and to the quality of personal relatedness, not cognitive structures *per se*; (iii) the theory gives weight to the role of the environmental object as a moderating factor in the development of mental and emotional life, but it also stipulates several mechanisms (pathological projective identification) by which the environmental object can be misused for defensive purposes; (iv) the theory contains a subtheory of anti-thinking and anti-knowing which attempts to clarify how emotional growth becomes defensively inhibited or reversed.

In Mel's case his 'mindlessness' took the form of a lack of differentiation between bodily and emotional levels of experience which allowed mental states and processes to be bypassed through the use of the body. Keeping painful emotions sequestered in his mind to do with his loss of and removal from his family led to their reappearance as 'lumps', which found such vivid expression through oral, phallic and anal themes. Once physical 'lumps' could be upgraded to the status of (i) a primitive *emotional* experience that required mental processing by a person, and (ii) a mental *concept* that through active verbalization by his therapist could beget a number of symbolic meanings, there could occur a diminution of impulsivity and acting out.

In the case of Brian, he fits the profile of a child with an 'organised introversion' (Winnicott 1952) – a boy whose emotional life was severely restricted by an arrangement of paranoid defences that ensured his feelings were buried in 'code', and that his object relations were characterized by a 'connecting-off' approach. This created special technical problems around making contact with him. A focus, however, by the therapist on the distinct anxieties around which these defensive formations had become encrusted brought forth the possibility of greater contact, especially with his teachers and his parents, who were better able to reach him with their didactic efforts.

Bibliography

Abraham, K. (1924) 'A short study of the development of the libido, viewed in the light of mental disorders' in *Selected Papers*, London: Hogarth Press.
—— (1927). *Selected Papers on Psychoanalysis*, London: Maresfield Reprints, 1979.
Adler, G. (1981) 'The borderline-narcissistic personality disorder continuum' *American Journal of Psychiatry* 138: 46–50.
—— (1985) *Borderline Psychopathology and its Treatment*, New York: Jason Aronson.
Ainsworth, M.D. (1985) 'Attachments across the lifespan' *Bulletin of the New York Academy of Medicine* 61: 792–812.
Ainsworth, M.D. and Bell, S.M. (1974) 'Mother–infant interaction and the development of competence' in K. Connolly and J. Bruner (eds) *The Growth of Competence*, New York: Academic Press.
Ainsworth, M.D., Blehar, M.C., Waters, E. and Wall, S. (1978) *Patterns of Attachment: A Psychological Study of the Strange Situation*, Hillsdale, NJ: Erlbaum.
Akiskal, H.S. (1981) 'Sub-affective disorders: dysthymic, cyclothymic and bipolar II disorders in the "borderline" realm' *Psychiatric Clinics of North America* 4: 25–46.
Alvarez, A. (1985) 'The problem of neutrality: some reflections on the psychoanalytic attitude in the treatment of borderline and psychotic children' *Journal of Child Psychotherapy* 11, 1: 87–103.
—— (1989) 'Development toward the latency period: splitting and the need to forget in borderline children' *Journal of Child Psychotherapy* 15, 2: 71–83.
—— (1992) *Live Company: Psychoanalytic Psychotherapy with Autistic, Borderline, Deprived and Abused Children*, London: Routledge.
—— (1997) 'Projective identification as a communication: its grammar in borderline psychotic children' *Psychoanalytic Dialogues* 7: 753–68.

American Psychiatric Association (1980) *Diagnostic and Statistical Manual of Mental Disorders* (3rd edn) Washington, DC: APA.

—— (1987) *Diagnostic and Statistical Manual of Mental Disorders* (3rd edn, revised) Washington, DC: APA.

—— (1994) *Diagnostic and Statistical Manual of Mental Disorders* (4th edn) Washington, DC: APA.

Andrulonis, P. (1991) 'Disruptive behavior disorders in boys and the borderline personality disorder in men' *Annals of Clinical Psychiatry* 3: 23–6.

Andrulonis, P., Glueck, B., Stroebel, C., Vogel, N., Shapiro, A. and Aldridge, D. (1981) 'Organic brain dysfunction and the borderline syndrome' *Psychiatric Clinics of North America* 4: 47–66.

Astington, J.W. (1994) *The Child's Discovery of the Mind*, London: Fontana Press.

Balint, M. (1969) 'Trauma and object relationship' *International Journal of Psychoanalysis* 50: 429–35.

Baron-Cohen, S. (1990) 'Autism: a specific cognitive disorder of "mind-blindness"' *International Review of Psychiatry* 2: 81–90.

—— (1995) *Mindblindness: An Essay on Autism and Theory of Mind*, Cambridge, MA, Bradford: MIT Press.

Bartsch, K. and Wellman, H.M. (1989) 'Young children's attribution of action to beliefs and desires' *Child Development* 60: 946–64.

Beeghly, M. and Cicchetti, D. (1994) 'Child maltreatment, attachment, and the self system: emergence of an internal state lexicon in toddlers at high social risk' *Development and Psychopathology* 6: 5–30.

Bemporad, J., Smith, H., Hanson, G. and Cicchetti, D. (1982) 'Borderline syndromes in childhood: criteria for diagnosis' *American Journal of Psychiatry* 139: 596–602.

Bick, E. (1968) 'The experience of the skin in early object-relations' *International Journal of Psychoanalysis* 49: 484–6.

Bion, W.R. (1957) 'Differentiation of the psychotic from the non-psychotic personalities' *International Journal of Psychoanalysis* 38: 266–75.

—— (1959) 'Attacks on linking' *International Journal of Psychoanalysis* 40: 308–15.

—— (1962a) *Learning from Experience*, London: Heinemann.

—— (1962b) 'A theory of thinking' *International Journal of Psychoanalysis* 43: 306–10.

—— (1967) *Second Thoughts*, New York: Jason Aronson.

Bleiberg, E. (1989) 'Stages of residential treatment: application of a developmental model' in J. Sanders (ed.) *Psychoanalytic Approaches to the Very Troubled Child*, New York: Haworth Press.

—— (1991) 'Mood disorders in children and adolescents' *Bulletin of the Menninger Clinic* 55: 182–204.

—— (1994) 'Borderline disorders in children and adolescents: the concept, the diagnosis, and the controversies' *Bulletin of the Menninger Clinic* 58, 2: 169–96.

Bleiberg, E., Fonagy, P. and Target, M. (1997) 'Child psychoanalysis: critical overview and a proposed reconsideration' *Psychiatric Clinics of North America* 6: 1–38.

Blum, H.P. (1974) 'The borderline childhood of the Wolfman' *Journal of the American Psychoanalytic Association* 22: 721–42.

Bolas, C. (1991) *The Forces of Destiny: Psychoanalysis and the Human Condition*, London: Free Association Books.

Bolton, D. and Hill, J. (1996) *Mind, Meaning and Mental Disorder*, Oxford: Oxford University Press.

Bowlby, J. (1969) *Attachment and Loss*, vol. 1: *Attachment*, London: Hogarth Press and The Institute of Psycho-Analysis.

—— (1973) *Attachment and Loss*, vol. 2: *Separation: Anxiety and Anger*. London: Hogarth Press and The Institute of Psycho-Analysis.

—— (1979) 'On knowing what you are not supposed to know and feeling what you are not supposed to feel' *Canadian Journal of Psychiatry* 24: 403–8.

Breier, A., Kelsoe, J., Kirwin, P., Beller, S., Wolkowitz, O. and Picka, D. (1988) 'Early parental loss and development of adult psychopathology' *Archives of General Psychiatry* 45: 987–93.

Brown, J.R. and Dunn, J. (1991) '"You can cry, mum": the social and developmental implications of talk about internal states' *British Journal of Developmental Psychology* 9: 237–57.

Bruner, J.S. (1968) *Processes of Cognitive Growth: Infancy*, Worcester, MA: Clark University Press.

Carlsson, E. and Sroufe, L.A. (1995) 'Contribution of attachment theory to developmental psychopathology' in D. Cicchetti and D.J. Cohen (eds) *Developmental Psychopathology*, vol. 1: *Theory and Methods*, New York: Wiley.

Chethik, M. (1980) 'The borderline child' in J. Noshpitz (ed.) *Basic Handbook of Child Psychiatry*, New York: Basic Books.

Chethik, M. and Fast, I. (1970) 'A function of fantasy in the borderline child' *American Journal of Orthopsychiatry* 40: 756–65.

Chu, J.A. (1998) 'Dissociative symptomatology in adult patients with histories of childhood physical and sexual abuse' in J.D. Bremner and C.R. Marmar (eds) *Trauma, Memory and Dissociation*, Progress in Psychiatry, 54. Washington, DC: American Psychiatric Press.

Chu, J. and Dill, D. (1990) 'Dissociative symptoms in relation to childhood physical and sexual abuse' *American Journal of Psychiatry* 147: 887–92.

Chused, J. (1995) 'The therapeutic action of psychoanalysis: abstinence and informative experiences' *Journal of the American Psychoanalytic*

Association 44, 4: 1047–71.

Cicchetti, D. and Barnett, D. (1991) 'Attachment organisation in preschool aged maltreated children' *Developmental Psychopathology* 3: 397–411.

Cicchetti, D. and Beeghly, M. (1987) 'Symbolic development in maltreated youngsters: an organizational perspective' in D. Cicchetti and M. Beeghly (eds) *Atypical Symbolic Development: New Directions for Child Development*, San Francisco: Jossey-Bass.

Cicchetti, D. and Cohen, D. (1995) *Developmental Psychopathology*, New York: Wiley Interscience.

Coates, S., Freidman, R.C. and Wolfe, S. (1991) 'The etiology of boyhood gender identity disorder: a model for integrating temperament, development and psychodynamics' *Psychoanalytic Dialogues* 1: 481–523.

Cohen, D.J., Paul, R. and Volkmar, F.R. (1986) 'Issues in the classification of pervasive and other developmental disorders: towards DSM IV' *Journal of the American Academy of Child Psychiatry* 25, 2: 213–20.

Cohen, D.J., Towbin, K.E., Mayes, L. and Volkmar, F. (1994) 'Developmental psychopathology of multicomplex disorder' in S.L. Freedman and H.C. Haywood (eds) *Developmental Follow-Up: Concepts, Genres, Domains and Methods*, New York: Academic Press.

Davidson, D. (1983) *Inquiries into Truth and Interpretation*, Oxford: Oxford University Press.

Delozier, P. (1982) 'Attachment theory and child abuse' in C.M. Parkes (ed.) *The Place of Attachment in Human Behaviour*, London: Basic Books.

Dennett, D.C. (1978) 'Beliefs about beliefs' *Behavioural and Brain Sciences* 4: 568–70.

Dias, M.G. and Harris, P.L. (1990) 'The influence of the imagination on reasoning by young children' *British Journal of Developmental Psychology* 8: 305–18.

Dickes, R. (1974) 'The concept of borderline states: an alternative proposal' *International Journal of Psychoanalytic Psychotherapy* 3: 1–27.

—— (1978) 'Parents, transitional objects and childhood fetishes' in S.A. Grolnick and L. Barkin (eds) *Between Reality and Fantasy*, New York: Jason Aronson.

Dunn, J. (1996) 'Children's relationships: bridging the divide between cognitive and social development', The Emanuel Miller Memorial Lecture 1995, *Journal of Child Psychology and Psychiatry* 37: 507–18.

Edgecombe, R. (1995) 'The history of Anna Freud's thinking on developmental disturbances' *Bulletin of the Anna Freud Centre* 18: 21–34.

Ekstein, R. (1966) *Children of Time and Space, of Action and Impulse*, New York: Appleton-Century-Crofts.

Ekstein, R. and Wallerstein, J. (1954) 'Observations on the psychology of borderline and psychotic children' *The Psychoanalytic Study of the Child* 9: 344–69.

—— (1956) 'Observations on the psychotherapy of borderline and psychotic children' *The Psychoanalytic Study of the Child* 11: 303–69.

—— (1957) 'Choice of interpretation in the treatment of borderline and psychotic children' *Bulletin of the Menninger Clinic* 21: 199–208.

Fairbairn, W.R.D. (1952) *Psychoanalytic Studies of the Personality*, London: Routledge and Kegan Paul.

Famularo, R., Kinscherff, R. and Fenton, T. (1991) 'Posttraumatic stress disorder among children clinically diagnosed as borderline personality disorder' *Journal of Nervous and Mental Disease* 179: 428–31.

Finkelhor, D. and Brown, A. (1985) 'The traumatic impact of childhood sexual abuse' *American Journal of Orthopsychiatry* 55: 530–41.

Finzy, R.T. (1971) 'Vicissitudes of the transitional object in a borderline child' *International Journal of Psychoanalysis* 52: 107–14.

Fischer, K.W., Kenny, S.L. and Pipp, S.L. (1990) 'How cognitive processes and environmental conditions organize discontinuities in the development of abstractions' in C.N. Alexander, E.J. Langer and R.M. Oetzel (eds) *Higher Stages of Development*, New York: Oxford University Press.

Fonagy, P. (1991) 'Thinking about thinking: some clinical and theoretical considerations in the treatment of a borderline patient' *International Journal of Psychoanalysis* 72: 639–55.

—— (1995) 'Playing and reality: the development of psychic reality and its malfunction in borderline personalities' *International Journal of Psychoanalysis* 76: 39–44.

Fonagy, P., Edgcumbe, R., Target, M., Miller, J. and Moran, G.S. (in press) *Contemporary Psychodynamic Child Therapy: Theory and Technique*, New York: Guilford Press.

Fonagy, P. and Higget, A. (1990) 'A developmental perspective on borderline personality disorder' *Revue Internationale de Psychopathologie* 1: 125–59.

Fonagy, P., Leigh, T., Steele, M., Steele, H., Kennedy, R., Mattoon, G. and Target, M. (1996) 'The relation of attachment status, psychiatric classification, and response to psychotherapy' *Journal of Consulting and Clinical Psychology* 64: 22–31.

Fonagy, P. and Moran, G.S. (1993) 'Childhood diabetes' in A.J. Solnit (ed.) *Textbook of Psychiatry*, Philadelphia: J.B. Lippincott.

Fonagy, P., Moran, G.S., Edgcumbe, R., Kennedy, H. and Target, M. (1993) 'The roles of mental representations and mental processes in therapeutic action' *The Psychoanalytic Study of the Child* 48: 9–48.

Fonagy, P., Moran, G.S., Kurtz, A., Bolton, A.M. and Brook, C. (1991) 'A controlled study of the psychoanalytic treatment of brittle diabetes' *Journal of the American Academy of Child Psychiatry* 30: 241–57.

Fonagy, P., Moran, G.S. and Target, M. (1993) 'Aggression and the psychological self' *International Journal of Psychoanalysis* 74: 471–85.

Fonagy, P., Redfern, S. and Charman, T. (1997) 'The relationship between belief-desire reasoning and a projective measure of attachment security (SAT)' *British Journal of Developmental Psychology* 15: 51–61.

Fonagy, P., Steele, H. and Holder, J. (submitted) 'Quality of attachment to mother at 1 year predicts belief-desire reasoning at 5 years' *Child Development*.

Fonagy, P., Steele, H., Moran, G., Steele, M. and Higgitt, A. (1991) 'The capacity for understanding mental states: the reflective self in parent and child and its significance for security of attachment' *Infant Mental Health Journal* 13: 200–17.

Fonagy, P., Steele, H. and Steele, M. (1991) 'Maternal representations of attachment during pregnancy predict the organization of infant–mother attachment at one year of age' *Child Development* 62: 891–905.

Fonagy, P., Steele, M., Steele, H., Higgitt, A. and Target, M. (1994) 'Theory and practice of resilience' *Journal of Child Psychology and Psychiatry* 35: 231–57.

Fonagy, P., Steele, M., Steele, H. and Target, M. (1997) 'Reflective-functioning manual, version 4.1, for application to Adult Attachment Interviews' Unpublished manuscript, University College London.

Fonagy, P. and Target, M. (1994) 'The efficacy of psychoanalysis for children with disruptive diabetes' *Journal of the American Academy of Child Psychiatry* 33: 45–55.

—— (1995) 'Towards understanding violence: the use of the body and the role of the father' *International Journal of Psychoanalysis* 76: 487–502.

—— (1996a) 'A contemporary psychoanalytic perspective: psycho-dynamic developmental therapy' in E. Hibbs and P. Jensen (eds) *Psychosocial Treatments for Child and Adolescent Disorders: Empirically Based Approaches*, Washington, DC: APA and NIH.

—— (1996b) 'Predictors of outcome in child psychoanalysis: a retrospective study of 763 cases at the Anna Freud Centre' *Journal of the American Psychoanalytic Association* 44: 27–77.

—— (1997) 'Attachment and reflective function: their role in self-organisation' *Development and Psychopathology* 9: 679–700.

Frank, H. and Paris, J. (1981) 'Recollections of family experience in borderline patients' *Archives of General Psychiatry* 38: 1031–4.

Freud, A. (1936) *The Ego and the Mechanisms of Defence*, London: Hogarth Press.

—— (1945) 'Indications for child analysis' in *The Writings of Anna Freud* 4: 3–38. New York: International Universities Press.

—— (1956) 'The assessment of borderline cases' in *The Writings of Anna Freud* 5: 301–14. New York: International Universities Press.

—— (1962) 'Assessment of childhood disturbances' *The Psychoanalytic Study of the Child* 17: 149–58.

—— (1965) 'Normality and pathology in childhood' in *The Writings of Anna Freud* 6. New York: International Universities Press.

Freud, S. (1905) 'Three essays on the theory of sexuality' S.E. 7: 135–243.

—— (1911a) 'Formulations on the two principles of mental functioning' S.E. 12: 218–26.

—— (1911b) 'Psychoanalytic notes on an autobiographical account of a case of paranoia' S.E. 12: 9–82.

—— (1914) 'On narcissism: an introduction' S.E. 14: 73–104.

—— (1924) 'The economic problem of masochism' S.E. 19: 159–70.

—— (1926) 'Inhibitions, symptoms and anxiety' S.E. 20: 87–174.

—— (1937) 'Analysis terminable and interminable' S.E. 23: 216–53.

—— (1938) 'Splitting of the ego in the process of defence' S.E. 23: 275–8.

Frijling-Schreuder, E. (1969) 'Borderline states in children' *The Psychoanalytic Study of the Child* 24: 307–27.

Furman, E. (1974) *A Child's Parent Dies: Studies in Childhood Bereavement*, New Haven, CT: Yale University Press.

Gabbard, G. (1994) *Psychodynamic Psychiatry in Clinical Practice: The DSM-IV Edition*, Washington, DC: American Psychiatric Press.

Gedo, J. and Gehrie, M.J. (1993) *Impasse and Innovation in Psychoanalysis*, Hillsdale, NJ: Analytic Press.

Geleerd, E.R. (1946) 'A contribution to the problem of psychosis in childhood' *The Psychoanalytic Study of the Child* 2: 271–93.

—— (1949) 'Psychoanalysis of a psychotic child' *The Psychoanalytic Study of the Child* 3/4: 311–32.

—— (1958) 'Borderline states in children and adolescents' *The Psychoanalytic Study of the Child* 13: 279–95.

Gergely, G. and Watson, J. (1996) 'The social biofeedback model of parental affect-mirroring' *International Journal of Psychoanalysis* 77: 1181–212.

Glenn, J. (1978) *Child Analysis and Therapy*, New York: Jason Aronson.

Goldberg, R., Mann, L., Wise, T. and Segall, E. (1985) 'Parental qualities as perceived by borderline personality disorders' *Journal of Clinical Psychiatry* 7: 134–40.

Goldman, S., D'Angelo, E. and DeMaso, D. (1993) 'Psychopathology in the families of children and adolescents with borderline personality disorder' *American Journal of Psychiatry* 150: 1832–5.

Goldman, S., D'Angelo, E., DeMaso, D. and Mezzacappa, E. (1992) 'Physical and sexual abuse histories among children with borderline personality disorder' *American Journal of Psychiatry* 149: 1723–6.

Goodwin, J., Cheeves, K. and Connell, V. (1990) 'Borderline and other severe symptoms in adult survivors of incestuous abuse' *Psychiatric Annals* 20: 22–4, 27–32.

Gopnik, A. (1993) 'How we know our minds: the illusion of first-person knowledge of intentionality' *Behavioural and Brain Sciences* 16: 1–14, 29–113.

Gopnik, A. and Astington, J.W. (1988) 'Children's understanding of representational change and its relation to the understanding of false belief and the appearance–reality distinction' *Child Development* 59: 26–37.

Greenacre, P. (1953) 'Certain relationships between fetishism and the faulty development of the body image' *The Psychoanalytic Study of the Child* 8: 79–98.

—— (1968) 'Perversions: general considerations regarding their genetic and dynamic background' *The Psychoanalytic Study of the Child* 23: 47–62.

—— (1979) 'Fetishism' in I. Rosen (ed.) *Sexual Deviations* (2nd edn), Oxford: Oxford University Press.

Greenspan, S.I. (1989) *The Development of the Ego in the Course of Life*, vol. 1: *Infancy*, Madison, CT: International Universities Press.

Grinker, R.R., Werble, B. and Drye, R.C. (1968) *The Borderline Syndrome: A Behavioural Study of Ego-Functions*, New York: Basic Books.

Grossman, K.E., Grossman, K. and Schwan, A. (1986) 'Capturing the wider view of attachment: a reanalysis of Ainsworth's Strange Situation' in C.E. Izard and P.B. Read (eds) *Measuring Emotions in Infants and Children*, New York: Cambridge University Press.

Grossman, K.E., Loher, I., Grossmann, K., Scheuerer-Englisch, H., Schildbach, B., Spangler, G., Wensauer, M. and Wimmermann, P. (1993) 'The development of inner working models of attachment and adaptation', Paper presented at the 60th Anniversary Meeting of the Society for Research in Child Development, New Orleans.

Grotstein, J. (1979) 'The psychoanalytic concept of the borderline organization' in J. LeBoit and A. Capponi (eds) *Advances in the Psychotherapy of the Borderline Patient*, London: Jason Aronson.

—— (1981) *Splitting and Projective Identification*, London: Jason Aronson.

Gunderson, J.G. (1984) *Borderline Personality Disorder*, Washington, DC: American Psychiatric Press.

Gunderson, J.G. and Singer, M.T. (1975) 'Defining borderline patients: an overview' *American Journal of Psychiatry* 132: 1–10.

Gunderson, J.G. and Zanarini, M.C. (1987) 'Current overview of the borderline diagnosis' *Journal of Clinical Psychiatry* 48 (Suppl.): 5–11.

—— (1989) 'Pathogenesis of borderline personality' in A. Tasman, R. Hales and A. Frances (eds) *American Psychiatric Press Review of Psychiatry*, Washington, DC: American Psychiatric Press.

Harris, P.L. (1994) 'The child's understanding of emotion: developmental change and the family environment' *Journal of Child Psychology and Psychiatry* 35: 3–28.

Harris, T., Brown, G. and Bifulco, A. (1986) 'Loss of parent in childhood and adult psychiatric disorder: the role of lack of adequate parental care' *Psychological Medicine* 16: 641–59.

Hedges, L.E. (1983) *Listening Perspectives in Psychotherapy*, London: Jason Aronson.

Heimann, P. (1952) 'Certain functions of introjection and projection in early infancy' in M. Klein, P. Heimann, S. Isaacs and J. Riviere (eds) *Developments in Psychoanalysis*, London: Hogarth Press.

Henry, G. (1974) 'Doubly deprived' *Journal of Child Psychotherapy* 4, 20: 29–43.

Herman, J. (1992) *Trauma and Recovery*, New York: Basic Books.

Herman, J., Perry, J. and Van der Kolk, B. (1989) 'Childhood trauma in borderline personality disorder' *American Journal of Psychiatry* 146: 490–5.

Hinshelwood, R.D. (1989) *A Dictionary of Kleinian Thought*, London: Free Association Books.

Hobson, R.P. (1986) 'The autistic child's appraisal of expressions of emotions' *Journal of Child Psychology and Psychiatry* 27, 3: 321–42.

—— (1993) *Autism and the Development of Mind*, Hillsdale, NJ: Erlbaum.

Hoffman, L. (1993) 'An introduction to child psychoanalysis' *Journal of Clinical Psychoanalysis* 2: 5–26.

Hopkins, J. (1977) 'Living under the threat of death' *Journal of Child Psychotherapy* 4: 5–22.

Hughes, A. (1988) 'The uses of manic defence in a 10-year-old girl' *International Review of Psychoanalysis* 15: 157–64.

Hurry, A. (1998) *Psychoanalysis and Developmental Therapy*, London: Karnac.

International Classification of Diseases 10 (1997) Geneva: WHO.

Isaacs, S. (1943) 'Acute psychotic anxiety occurring in a boy of 4 years' *International Journal of Psychoanalysis* 24: 13–32.

Jackson, J. (1970) 'Child psychotherapy in a school for maladjusted children' *Journal of Child Psychotherapy* 2, 4: 54–62.

—— (1985) 'An adolescent's difficulty in using his mind: some technical problems' *Journal of Child Psychotherapy* 11: 105–19.

Jacobson, E. (1964) *The Self and the Object World*, New York: International Universities Press.

Joseph, B. (1978) 'Different kinds of anxiety and their handling in the clinical situation' in M. Feldman and E. Spillius (eds) *Psychic Equilibrium and Psychic Change*, London: Tavistock/Routledge.

—— (1981) 'Defense mechanisms and phantasy in the psychoanalytic process' *Bulletin of the European Psychoanalytic Federation* 17: 11–24.

—— (1983) 'On understanding and not understanding: some technical issues' in M. Feldman and E. Spillius (eds) *Psychic Equilibrium and Psychic Change*, London: Tavistock/Routledge, 1989.

—— (1987) 'Projective identification: some clinical aspects' in M. Feldman and E. Spillius (eds) *Psychic Equilibrium and Psychic Change*, London: Tavistock/Routledge, 1989.

Kagan, J. (1994) *Galen's Prophecy*, New York: Basic Books.

Kandel, E. (1983) 'From metapsychology to molecular biology: explorations into the nature of anxiety' *American Journal of Psychiatry* 140: 1277–93.

Kernberg, O. (1967) 'Borderline personality organization' *Journal of the American Psychoanalytic Association* 15: 641–85.

—— (1975) *Borderline Conditions and Pathological Narcissism*, New York: Jason Aronson.

Kernberg, P. (1983a) 'Borderline conditions: childhood and adolescent aspects' in K. Robson (ed.) *The Borderline Child*, New York: McGraw-Hill.

—— (1983b) 'Issues in the psychotherapy of borderline conditions in children' in K. Robson (ed.) *The Borderline Child*, New York: McGraw-Hill.

—— (1994) 'Mechanisms of defense: development and research perspectives' *Bulletin of the Menninger Clinic* 58, 1: 55–87.

—— (1995) 'Child psychiatry: individual psychotherapy' in H. Kaplan and J. Sadock (eds) *Comprehensive Textbook of Psychiatry* (6th edn), Baltimore, MD: Williams and Wilkins.

Kernberg, P. and Shapiro, T. (1990) 'Resolved: borderline personality exists in children under twelve' (Debate forum: Affirmative and affirmative rebuttal) *American Academy of Child and Adolescent Psychiatry* 29: 478–82.

Kestenbaum, C. (1983) 'The borderline child at risk for major psychiatric disorder in adult life: seven case reports with follow-up' in K. Robson (ed.) *The Borderline Child*, New York: McGraw-Hill.

Khan, M.M.R. (1972) 'Exorcism of intrusive ego-alien factors in the analytic situation and process' in *The Privacy of the Self*, London: Hogarth Press.

Klein, D. (1977) 'Psychopharmacological treatment and delineation of borderline disorders' in P. Hartocollis (ed.) *Borderline Personality Disorders*, New York: International Universities Press.

Klein, M. (1923) 'The role of school in the libidinal development of the child' in *The Writings of Melanie Klein*, vol. 1, London: Hogarth Press, 1975.

—— (1930a) 'The importance of symbol-formation in the development of the ego' in *The Writings of Melanie Klein*, vol. 1, London: Hogarth Press, 1975.

—— (1930b) 'The psychotherapy of the psychoses' in *The Writings of Melanie Klein*, vol. 1, London: Hogarth Press, 1975.

—— (1932) 'The psychoanalysis of children' in *The Writings of Melanie Klein*, vol. 2, London: Hogarth Press, 1975.

—— (1935) 'A contribution to the psychogenesis of manic-depressive states' in *The Writings of Melanie Klein*, vol. 1, London: Hogarth Press, 1975.

—— (1940) 'Mourning and its relation to manic-depressive states' in *The Writings of Melanie Klein*, vol. 1, London: Hogarth Press, 1975.

—— (1946) 'Notes on some schizoid mechanisms' *International Journal of Psychoanalysis* 27: 99–110.

—— (1952) 'Some theoretical conclusions regarding the emotional life of the infant' in *The Writings of Melanie Klein*, vol. 3, London: Hogarth Press, 1975.

Kohut, H. (1977) *The Restoration of the Self*, New York: International Universities Press.

Laplanche, J. and Pontalis, B. (1973) *The Language of Psychoanalysis*, London: Hogarth Press.

LeBoit, J. and Capponi, A. (1979) 'The technical problem with the borderline patient' in J. BeBoit and A. Capponi (eds) *Advances in the Psychotherapy of the Borderline Patient*, London: Jason Aronson.

Leichtman, M. and Nathan, S. (1983) 'A clinical approach to the psychological testing of borderline children' in K. Robson (ed.) *The Borderline Child*, New York: McGraw-Hill.

Levinson, A. and Fonagy, P. (submitted) 'Attachment classification in prisoners and psychiatric patients' *British Journal of Psychiatry*.

Linehan, M. (1993) *Cognitive Behavioral Treatment of Borderline Personality*, New York: Guilford Press.

Little, M. (1981) *Transference Neurosis and Transference Psychosis*, New York and London: Jason Aronson.

Lofgren, D.P., Bemporad, J., King, J., Lindem, K. and O'Driscoll, G. (1991) 'A prospective follow-up study of so-called borderline children' *American Journal of Psychiatry* 11: 1541–7.

Lubbe, T. (1986) 'Some disturbed pupils' perceptions of their teachers: a psychotherapist's viewpoint' *Maladjustment and Therapeutic Education* 4, 1: 29–35.

Lush, D. (1968) 'Progress of a child with atypical development' *Journal of Child Psychotherapy* 2, 2: 64.

McParlane, A., Weber, D. and Clark, R. (1993) 'Abnormal stimulus processing in posttraumatic stress disorder' *Biological Psychiatry* 34: 311–20.

Mahler, M. (1952) 'On child psychosis and schizophrenia: autistic and symbiotic infantile psychosis' *The Psychoanalytic Study of the Child* 7: 286–305.

—— (1971) 'A study of the separation–individuation process: and its possible application to borderline phenomena in the psychoanalytical situation' *The Psychoanalytic Study of the Child* 26: 403–24.

Mahler, M., Pine, F. and Bergman, A. (1975) *The Psychological Birth of the Human Infant: Symbiosis and Individuation*, New York: Basic Books.

Mahler, M., Ross, J. and DeFries, Z. (1949) 'Clinical studies in benign and malignant cases of childhood psychoses' *American Journal of Orthopsychiatry* 19: 295–305.

Main, M. (1991) 'Metacognitive knowledge, metacognitive monitoring, and singular (coherent) vs multiple (incoherent) model of attachment: findings and directions for future research' in C.M. Parkes, J. Stevenson-Hinde and P. Marris (eds) *Attachment across the Life Cycle*, London: Tavistock/Routledge.

Main, M. and Hesse, E. (1990) 'Parents' unresolved traumatic experiences are related to infant disorganized attachment status: is frightened and/or frightening parental behavior the linking mechanism?' in M. Greenberg, D. Cicchetti and E.M. Cummings (eds) *Attachment in the Preschool Years: Theory, Research and Intervention*, Chicago: University of Chicago Press.

Main, M. and Solomon, J. (1990) 'Procedures for identifying infants as disorganized/disoriented during the Ainsworth Strange Situation' in M. Greenberg, D. Cicchetti and E.M. Cummings (eds) *Attachment in the Preschool Years: Theory, Research and Intervention*, Chicago: University of Chicago Press.

Marcus, J. (1963) 'Borderline states in childhood' *Journal of Child Psychoanalytic Psychiatry* 4: 208–18.

Marohn, R. (1991) 'Psychotherapy of adolescents with behavioral disorders' in M. Slomowitz (ed.) *Adolescent Psychotherapy*, Washington, DC: American Psychiatric Press.

Marohn, R., Offer, D., Ostrov, E. and Trujillo, J. (1979) 'Four psychodynamic types of hospitalized juvenile delinquents' *Adolescent Psychiatry* 7: 466–83.

Massie, H.N. and Rosenthal, J. (1984) *Child Psychosis in the First Four Years of Life*, New York: McGraw-Hill.

Masterson, J. (1972) *Treatment of the Borderline Adolescent: A Developmental Approach*, New York: John Wiley.

Masterson, J. and Rinsley, D. (1975) 'The borderline syndrome: the role of the mother in the genesis and psychic structure of the borderline personality' *International Journal of Psychoanalysis* 56: 163–77.

Meltzer, D. (1967) *The Psychoanalytical Process*, Strath Tay: Clunie Press.

—— (1973) *Sexual States of Mind*, Strath Tay: Clunie Press.

—— (1986) *Studies in Extended Metapsychology*, Strath Tay: Clunie Press.

Meltzer, D., Bremner, J., Hoxter, S., Wedell, H. and Wittenberg, I. (1975) *Explorations in Autism*, Strath Tay: Clunie Press.

Mitchell, S. (1988) *Relational Concepts in Psychoanalysis*, Cambridge, MA: Harvard University Press.

Modell, A.H. (1963) 'Primitive object relationships, predisposition to schizophrenia' *International Journal of Psychoanalysis* 44: 282–92.

Money-Kyrle, R. (1977) 'On being a psychoanalyst' in D. Meltzer and E. O'Shaugnessey (eds) *The Collective Papers of Roger Money-Kyrle*, Strath Tay: Clunie Press.

Moore, B.E. and Fine, P.C. (1968) *Glossary of Psychoanalytic Terms and Concepts*, New York: American Psychoanalytic Association.

Moran, G.S. (1984) 'Psychoanalytic treatment of diabetic children' *The Psychoanalytic Study of the Child* 38: 265–93.

Morton, J. and Frith, U. (1995) 'Causal modelling: a structural approach to developmental psychology' in D. Cicchetti and D.J. Cohen (eds) *Developmental Psychopathology*, vol. 1: *Theory and Methods*, New York: John Wiley.

Murburgh, M. (1994) *Catecholamine Function in Posttraumatic Stress Disorder: Emerging Concepts*, Washington, DC: American Psychiatric Press.

Nagera, H. (1970) 'Children's reactions to the death of important objects: a developmental approach' *The Psychoanalytic Study of the Child* 25: 360–400.

Offer, D., Marohn, R. and Ostrov, E. (1979) *The Psychological World of the Juvenile Delinquent*, New York: Basic Books.

Ogata, S., Silk, K. and Goodrich, S. (1990) 'The childhood experiences of the borderline patient' in P. Links (ed.) *Family Environment and the Borderline Patient*, Washington, DC: American Psychiatric Press.

Ornstein, P.H. (1983) 'Discussion of papers by Drs Goldberg, Stolorow and Wallerstein' in J.D. Lichtenberg and S. Kaplan (eds) *Reflections of Self Psychology*, London: Analytic Press.

Pamularo, R., Kinscherff, R. and Fenton, J. (1991) 'Post-traumatic stress disorder among children clinically diagnosed as borderline personality' *Journal of Nervous and Mental Disorders* 179: 428–31.

Paris, J. and Frank, H. (1989) 'Perceptions of parental bonding in borderline patients' *American Journal of Psychiatry* 146: 1498–9.

Paris, J. and Zweig-Frank, H. (1992) 'A critical review of the role of childhood sexual abuse in the etiology of borderline personality disorder' *Canadian Journal of Psychiatry* 37: 125–8.

—— (1997) 'Parameters of childhood sexual abuse in female patients' in M.C. Zanarini (ed.) *Role of Sexual Abuse in the Etiology of Borderline Personality Disorder*, Washington, DC: American Psychiatric Press.

Perner, J., Leekman, S. and Wimmer, H. (1987) 'Three-year-olds' difficulty in understanding false belief: cognitive limitation, lack of knowledge, or pragmatic misunderstanding?' *British Journal of Developmental Psychology* 5: 125–37.

Perner, J., Ruffman, T. and Leekman, S.R. (1994) 'Theory of mind is contagious: you catch it from your sibs' *Child Development* 65: 1228–38.

Perry, B. (1997) 'Incubated in terror: neurodevelopmental factors in the "cycle of violence"' in J. Osofsky (ed.) *Children in a Violent Society*, New York: Guilford Press.

Petot, J.-M. (1990) *Melanie Klein*, vol. 1: *First Discoveries and First Systems*, Madison, CT: International Universities Press.

Petti, T.A. and Vela, R.M. (1990) 'Borderline disorders of childhood: an overview' *Journal of the American Academy of Child and Adolescent Psychiatry* 29, 3: 327–37.

Pine, F. (1974) 'On the concept "borderline" in children' *The Psychoanalytic Study of the Child* 29: 341–68.

—— (1976) 'On therapeutic change: perspectives from a parent–child model' *Psychoanalysis and Contemporary Science* 4: 537–69.

—— (1983) 'A working nosology of borderline syndromes in children' in K. Robson (ed.) *The Borderline Child*, New York: McGraw-Hill.

Putnam, F. and Trickett, P. (1997) 'Psychobiological effects of sexual abuse: a longitudinal study' in R. Yehuda and A. McFarlane (eds) *Psychobiology of Posttraumatic Stress Disorder*, New York: New York Academy of Sciences.

Pynoos, R., Frederick, C., Nader, K., Arroyo, W., Steinberg, A., Eth, S., Nunez, F. and Fairbanks, L. (1987) 'Life threat and posttraumatic states in school-age children' *Archives of General Psychiatry* 44: 1057–63.

Rapoport, J.L. and Ismond, D.K. (1984) *DSM III Training Guide for Diagnosis of Childhood Disorders*, New York: Bruner/Masel.

Reid, S. (1990) 'The importance of beauty in the psychoanalytic experience' *Journal of Child Psychotherapy* 16: 29–52.

Renvoize, J. (1982) *Incest: A Family Pattern*, London: Routledge and Kegan Paul.

Rey, J.H. (1979) 'Schizoid phenomena in the borderline' in J. LeBoit and A. Capponi (eds) *Advances in the Psychotherapy of the Borderline Patient*, New York: Jason Aronson.

Rinsley, D. (1980) 'Diagnosis and treatment of borderline and narcissistic children and adolescents' *Bulletin of the Menninger Clinic* 44, 2: 147–70.

—— (1984) 'A comparison of borderline and narcissistic personality disorders' *Bulletin of the Menninger Clinic* 48: 1–9.

—— (1989) *Developmental Pathogenesis and Psychoanalytic Treatment of Borderline and Narcissistic Personalities*, Northvale, NJ: Jason Aronson.

Rosen, V.H. (1955) 'The reconstruction of a traumatic childhood event in a case of derealisation' *Journal of the American Psychoanalytic Association* 3: 211–21.

Rosenfeld, H. (1964) 'On the psychopathology of narcissism: a clinical approach' *International Journal of Psychoanalysis* 45: 332–7.

—— (1965) *Psychotic States: A Psychoanalytical Approach*, London: Hogarth Press.

—— (1987) *Impasse and Interpretation*, London: Tavistock.

Rosenfeld, S. (1972) 'Notes on self and object differentiation and communication in borderline children' in *Beyond the Infantile Neurosis*, London: Hampstead Clinic.

—— (1975) 'Some reflections arising from the treatment of a traumatised child' in *Hampstead Clinic Studies in Child Psychoanalysis. 20th Anniversary Proceedings*, New Haven: Yale University Press.

Rosenfeld, S. and Sprince, M. (1963) 'An attempt to formulate the meaning of the concept "borderline"' *The Psychoanalytic Study of the Child* 18: 603–35.

—— (1965) 'Some thoughts on the technical handling of borderline children' *The Psychoanalytic Study of the Child* 20: 495–517.

Sandler, J. (1962) 'The Hampstead Index as an instrument of psychoanalytic research' *International Journal of Psychoanalysis* 43: 287–91.

Sandler, J. with Freud, A. (1985) *The Analysis of Defence*, New York: International Universities Press.

Sandler, J., Kennedy, H. and Tyson, R. (1980) *The Technique of Child Analysis: Discussions with Anna Freud*, London: Hogarth Press.

Schimmer, R. (1983) 'The borderline personality organization in elementary school: conflict and treatment' in K. Robson (ed.) *The Borderline Child*, New York: McGraw-Hill.

Schneider-Rosen, K. and Cicchetti, D. (1984) 'The relationship between affect and cognition in maltreated infants: quality of attachment and the development of visual self-recognition' *Child Development* 55: 648–58.

—— (1991) 'Early self-knowledge and emotional development: visual self-recognition and affective reactions to mirror self-image in maltreated and non-maltreated toddlers' *Developmental Psychology* 27: 481–8.

Schore, A.N. (1996) 'The experience-dependent maturation of a regulatory system in the orbital prefrontal cortex and the origin of developmental psychopathology' *Development and Psychopathology* 8: 59–87.

Segal, H. (1957) 'Notes on symbol formation' *International Journal of Psychoanalysis* 38: 391–7.

—— (1979) *Klein*, London: Fontana/Collins.

Settlage, C.F. (1977) 'The psychoanalytic understanding of narcissistic and borderline personality disorders: advances in developmental theory' *Journal of the American Psychoanalytic Association* 25, 4: 805–33.

Shalev, A., Orr, S. and Pitman, R. (1993) 'Psychophysiologic assessment of traumatic imagery in Israeli civilian patients with posttraumatic stress disorders' *American Journal of Psychiatry* 150: 620–4.

Shapiro, T. (1979) 'Psychoanalytic classification and empiricism with borderline personality disorder as a model' *Journal of Consulting and Clinical Psychology* 57, 2: 187–94.

—— (1983) 'The borderline syndrome in childhood: a critique' in K. Robson (ed.) *The Borderline Child*, New York: McGraw-Hill.

—— (1990) 'Resolved: borderline personality exists in children under twelve' (Debate forum: Affirmative and affirmative rebuttal) *American Academy of Child and Adolescent Psychiatry* 29: 478–82.

Sherick, I., Kearney, C., Buxtom, M. and Stevens, B. (1978) 'Ego strengthening psychotherapy with children having primary ego deficiencies' *Journal of Child Psychotherapy* 4, 4: 51–64.

Sinason, V. (1992) *Mental Handicap and the Human Condition*, London: Free Association Books.

Spillius, E. (1988) *Melanie Klein Today Vol. 2: Mainly Practice, Introduction*, London: Routledge.

Sroufe, L.A. (1983) *Infant–Caregiver Attachment and Patterns of Adaptation in Preschool: The Roots of Maladaption and Competence*, vol. 16. Hillsdale, NJ: Erlbaum.

—— (1988) 'The role of infant–caregiver attachment in development' in J. Belsky and T. Nezworski (eds) *Clinical Implications of Attachment: Child Psychology*, Hillsdale, NJ: Erlbaum.

—— (1996) *Emotional Development: The Organization of Emotional Life in the Early Years*, New York: Cambridge University Press.

Sroufe, L.A., Egeland, B. and Kreutzer, T. (1990) 'The fate of early experience following developmental change: longitudinal approaches to individual adaptation in childhood' *Child Development* 61: 1363–73.

Steele, M., Fonagy, P., Yabsley, S., Woolgar, M. and Croft, C. (1995) 'Maternal representations of attachment during pregnancy predict quality of children's doll play at 5 years of age', Paper presented to Society for Research in Child Development, Indianapolis.

Steele, H., Steele, M. and Fonagy, P. (1996) 'Associations among attachment classifications of mothers, fathers, and their infants: evidence for
a relationship-specific perspective' *Child Development* 67: 541–55.

Steiner, J. (1979) 'The border between the paranoid-schizoid and the
depressive positions in the borderline patient' *British Journal of
Medical Psychology* 52: 385–91.

—— (1987) 'The interplay between pathological organizations and the
paranoid-schizoid and the depressive positions' *International Journal
of Psychoanalysis* 68: 69–80.

—— (1991) 'A psychotic organization of the personality' *International
Journal of Psychoanalysis* 72: 201–7.

—— (1994) 'Patient-centered and analyst-centered interpretations: some
implications of containment and countertransference' *Psychoanalytic
Inquiry* 14: 406–22.

Stern, D.N. (1985) *The Interpersonal World of the Infant: A View from
Psychoanalysis and Developmental Psychology*, New York: Basic
Books.

Stone, M. (1979) 'Contemporary shift of the borderline concept from a
sub-schizophrenic disorder to a sub-affective disorder' *Psychiatric
Clinics of North America* 2: 577–94.

—— (1990) 'Abuse and abusiveness in borderline personality disorder'
in P. Links (ed.) *Family Environment and Borderline Personality
Disorder*, Washington, DC: American Psychiatric Press.

Stone, M., Kahn, E. and Flye, B. (1981) 'Psychiatrically ill relatives of
borderline patients: a family study' *Psychiatric Quarterly* 53: 71–84.

Stoller, R.J. (1975) *Perversion: The Erotic Form of Hatred*, New York:
Delta.

Stroh, G. (1974) 'Psychotic children' in P. Barker (ed.) *The Residential
Psychiatric Treatment of Children*, London: Crosby.

Suomi, S. (1987) 'Genetic and maternal contributions to individual
differences in rhesus monkey biobehavioral development' in
N. Krasnegor, E. Blass and M. Hofer (eds) *Perinatal Development:
A Psychobiological Perspective*, Orlando, FL: Academic Press.

—— (1992) 'Uptight and laid-back monkeys: individual differences in
behavioral development', Plenary presentation at the annual meeting
of the American Academy of Child and Adolescent Psychiatry,
Washington, DC.

Symington, N. (1983) 'The analyst's act of freedom as agent of therapeutic change' *International Review of Psychoanalysis* 10: 783–92.

Szur, R. (1983) 'Sexuality and aggression as related themes' in M. Boston
and R. Szur (eds) *Psychotherapy with Severely Deprived Children*
London: Routledge and Kegan Paul.

Target, M. (1993) 'The outcome of child psychoanalysis: a retrospective
investigation' Unpublished doctoral thesis, University of London.

Target, M. and Fonagy, P. (1994a) 'The efficacy of psychoanalysis for children with emotional disorders' *Journal of the American Academy of Child and Adolescent Psychiatry* 33: 361–71.

—— (1994b) 'The efficacy of psychoanalysis for children: developmental considerations' *Journal of the American Academy of Child and Adolescent Psychiatry* 33: 1134–44.

—— (1996) 'Playing with reality II: The development of psychic reality from a theoretical perspective' *International Journal of Psychoanalysis* 77: 459–79.

Tarnopolsky, A., Chesterman, P.C. and Parshall, A.M. (1995) 'What is psychosis?' *Free Associations* 5, 4: 536–66.

Terr, L. (1991) 'Childhood traumas: an outline and overview' *American Journal of Psychiatry* 148: 10–20.

—— (1994) *Unchained Memories: True Stories of Traumatic Memories, Lost and Found*, New York: Basic Books.

Tonnesmann, M. (1980) 'Adolescent re-enactment, trauma and reconstruction' *Journal of Child Psychotherapy* 6: 23–44.

Tooley, K. (1973) 'Playing it right – a technique for the treatment of borderline children' *Journal of the American Academy of Child Psychiatry* 12: 615–31.

Towbin, K.E., Dykens, E.M., Pearson, G.S. and Cohen, D.J. (1993) 'Conceptualizing "borderline syndrome of childhood" and "childhood schizophrenia" as a developmental disorder' *Journal of the Academy of Child and Adolescent Psychiatry* 32: 775–82.

Trowell, J. (1981) 'Psychosis or communication? The experience of chaos in a 4 year old girl' *Journal of Child Psychotherapy* 7: 47–57.

Tustin, F. (1972) *Autism and Childhood Psychosis*, London: Hogarth Press.

—— (1978) 'Psychotic elements in the neurotic disorders of children' *Journal of Child Psychotherapy* 4: 4: 5–17.

—— (1981) *Autistic States in Children*, London: Routledge.

—— (1988) 'Psychotherapy with children who cannot play' *International Review of Psychoanalysis* 15: 93–105.

Van der Kolk, B. (1989) 'The compulsion to repeat the trauma: re-enactment, re-victimization, and masochism' *Psychiatric Clinics of North America* 12: 389–411.

—— (1994) 'The body keeps the score: memory and the evolving psychobiology of post-traumatic stress' *Harvard Review of Psychiatry* 1: 253–65.

Van der Kolk, B. and Fisler, R. (1994) 'Childhood abuse and neglect and loss of self-regulation' *Bulletin of the Menninger Clinic* 58: 145–68.

Van der Kolk, B.A., Burbridge, J.A. and Suzuki, J. (1997) 'The psychobiology of traumatic memory' in R. Yehuda and A.C. McFarlane (eds)

Psychobiology of Post-traumatic Stress Disorder, Annals of the New York Academy of Sciences, vol. 821, New York: New York Academy of Sciences.

Van Reeum, R., Link, P. and Boigao, I. (1993) 'Constitutional factors in borderline personality disorder: genetics, brain dysfunction and biological markers' in J. Paris (ed.) *Borderline Personality Disorder: Etiology and Treatment*, Washington, DC: American Psychiatric Press.

Vela, R.M. Gottlieb, E.H. and Gottlieb, H.P. (1983) 'Borderline syndrome in childhood: a critical review' in K. Robson (ed.) *The Borderline Child: Approaches to Etiology, Diagnosis and Treatment*, New York: McGraw-Hill.

Waters, E., Wippman, J. and Sroufe, L.A. (1979) 'Attachment, positive affect, and competence in the peer group: two studies in construct validation' *Child Development* 50: 821–9.

Weil, A.P. (1953a) 'Certain severe disturbances of ego development in childhood' *The Psychoanalytic Study of the Child* 8: 271–87.

—— (1953b) 'Clinical data and dynamic considerations in certain cases of childhood schizophrenia' *American Journal of Orthopsychiatry* 23.

—— (1956) 'Some evidences of deviational development in infancy and early childhood' *The Psychoanalytic Study of the Child* 11: 292–9.

—— (1970) 'The basic core' *The Psychoanalytic Study of the Child* 25: 442–60.

Wender, P. (1977) 'The contribution of the adoption studies to an understanding of the phenomenology and etiology of borderline schizophrenia' in P. Hartocollis (ed.) *Borderline Personality Disorders: The Concept, the Syndrome, the Patient*, New York: International Universities Press.

Westen, D. (1990) 'Toward a revised theory of borderline object relations: implications of empirical research' *International Journal of Psychoanalysis* 71: 661–93.

Widiger, T.A., Miele, G.M. and Tilley, S.M. (1992) 'Alternative perspectives on the diagnosis of borderline personality disorder' in J.F. Clarkin, E. Marziali and H. Munroe-Blum (eds) *Borderline Personality Disorder: Clinical and Empirical Perspectives*, New York: Guilford Press.

Winnicott, D.W. (1952) 'Psychosis and child care' in *Through Pediatrics to Psychoanalysis*, London: Hogarth Press.

—— (1953) 'Transitional objects and transitional phenomena: a study of the first not-me possession' *International Journal of Psychoanalysis* 34: 89–97.

—— (1960a) 'Ego distortion in terms of true and false self' in *The Maturational Processes and the Facilitating Environment*, London: Hogarth Press.

—— (1960b) 'The theory of the parent–infant relationship' in *The Maturational Processes and the Facilitating Environment,* London: Hogarth Press.

—— (1965) *The Maturational Processes and the Facilitating Environment,* London: Hogarth Press.

—— (1967a) 'The concept of clinical regression compared with that of defense organization' in *Psychoanalytic Explorations,* London: Karnac Books.

—— (1967b) 'Mirror-role of mother and family in child development' in P. Lomas (ed.) *The Predicament of the Family,* London: Hogarth Press.

—— (1968) 'The use of an object and relating through identifications' in *Psychoanalytic Explorations,* London: Karnac Books.

—— (1969) 'Development of the theme of the mother's unconscious as discovered in psychoanalytic practice' in *Psychoanalytic Explorations,* London: Karnac Books.

—— (1971) *Playing and Reality,* London: Tavistock Publications.

—— (1985) 'The psychotherapy of character disorders' in C. Winnicott and M. Davis (eds) *Deprivation and Delinquency,* London: Tavistock/Routledge.

Wolfenstein, M. (1966) 'How is mourning possible?' *The Psychoanalytic Study of the Child* 21: 93–123.

Woods, J. (1982) 'Working towards interpretation: early stages in the treatment of a borderline psychotic boy' *Journal of Child Psychotherapy* 8, 2: 151.

—— (1985) 'Individual treatment needs in the therapeutic environment of a special school' *Journal of Child Psychotherapy* 11, 1: 51–65.

Yehuda, R. (1997) 'Sensitization of the hypothalamic–pituitary–adrenal axis in posttraumatic stress disorder' in R. Yehuda and A. McFarlane (eds) *Psychobiology of Posttraumatic Stress Disorder,* New York: New York Academy of Sciences.

Zanarini, M., Gunderson, J., Marino, M., Schwartz, E. and Frankenburg, F. (1989) 'Childhood experiences of borderline patients' *Comparative Psychiatry* 30: 18–25.

Zanarini, M.C. and Frankenburg, F.R. (1997) 'Pathways to the development of borderline personality disorder' *Journal of Personality Disorder* 11, 1: 93–104.

Zavitzianos, G. (1971) 'Fetishism and exhibitionism in the female and their relationship to psychopathy and kleptomania' *International Journal of Psychoanalysis* 52: 297–305.

Zweig-Frank, H. and Paris, J. (1997) 'Relationship of childhood sexual abuse to dissociation and self-mutilation in female patients' in M. Zanarini (ed.) *Role of Sexual Abuse in the Etiology of Borderline Personality Disorder,* Washington, DC: American Psychiatric Press.

Index